How Long Does it take,

To make,

A Fat Person?

And the secret to losing weight permanently in your lifetime.

Nehal Kaur

Dedication

With profound reverence, this volume is warmly dedicated to my beloved grandmother, the inaugural storyteller who gently wove historical narratives into my world. Her tales, transcending mere recollections, blossomed as seeds of inspiration within me, kindling an impassioned quest to explore the rich, layered annals of history. Her stories, whispered from a place of wisdom and experience, became a bridge to bygone eras, igniting a flame that illuminated my path through the intricate mazes of the past.

Moreover, this work is a heartfelt homage to the historians, scribes, and translators spanning across nations and epochs, who have generously bestowed upon us a legacy, rich and enlightening, enabling our journey through the magnificent tapestry of human history. These dedicated individuals, through their scrupulous writings and meticulous preservation of manuscripts, have safeguarded the threads of our collective past, allowing us to weave them into our present and future narratives. Their endeavors, often crafted in the silent alcoves of contemplation and research, have illuminated our path through history, and to them, we extend our deepest respect and eternal gratitude. May this work echo their diligence and stand as a testament to the unbreakable chain of stories that link us all through time.

CONTENTS

Acknowledgement

The reflections, insights, and knowledge articulated within these pages are deeply rooted in the wisdom and stories generously shared by my grandmother. Her narratives have not only shaped my understanding of history but have also kindled a flame of curiosity and reverence towards our collective past.

A heartfelt acknowledgment is extended to the British Broadcasting Corporation (BBC), whose enthralling history documentaries have been a staple of my childhood and a pivotal source of inspiration. The compelling storytelling and meticulous research evident in their productions ignited my desire to delve into the study of history and explore the myriad of books that have informed this work, many of which are cited in my bibliography.

A sincere thank you to all the authors and scholars mentioned therein. While I may not have traversed the entirety of your work, I have endeavoured to ensure that any direct quotations have been duly credited. Your contributions to the field have been instrumental in shaping this book and the broader understanding of our shared history.

I would also like to acknowledge KDP on this occasion, after over 50 years of being a sponge for all things historic, I have been prolific in recent months since discovering this platform. I had given up on the idea of ever publishing any of my half-finished manuscripts with a feeling of resignation that writing and publishing was the preserve of the well to do, and independently wealthy, so thank you KDP.

Introduction

I must declare upfront that my thesis posits that you possess as much control over whether you are a fat individual or a slim one as you do over whether you have the natural disposition to become a powerful, muscular Olympic standard one-hundred-meter sprinter or, conversely, a lean, svelte Olympic long-distance marathon runner.

In this book, I aim to share my empirical observations gleaned from studying the history of virtually every cultural and ethnic group, in the world. My conclusion is that genetics largely determines your body size and shape, shaped over generations by exposure to your environment and the abundance of food therein. I will elucidate the predisposition to human body size, shape, and body fat mass index — approximately 70% predetermined by genes versus 30% influenced by dietary discipline and lifestyle, according to my theory. This argument will be supported by statistical studies, empirical evidence, and simplified explanations on how our genes are the overarching determining factor. While there will be some disheartening news for many, the final chapters will bring some encouraging insights.

Statistics reveal that the United States has the largest proportion of obese individuals as a percentage of its population, a phenomenon that has developed over the past 250 years. The general populace of the US is predominantly composed of immigrants who migrated from famine-stricken countries such as Ireland and other similarly impoverished regions in Europe. My thesis suggests that these individuals were not overweight to begin with. However, as a species, humans have had to adapt to an environment with an overabundance of food.

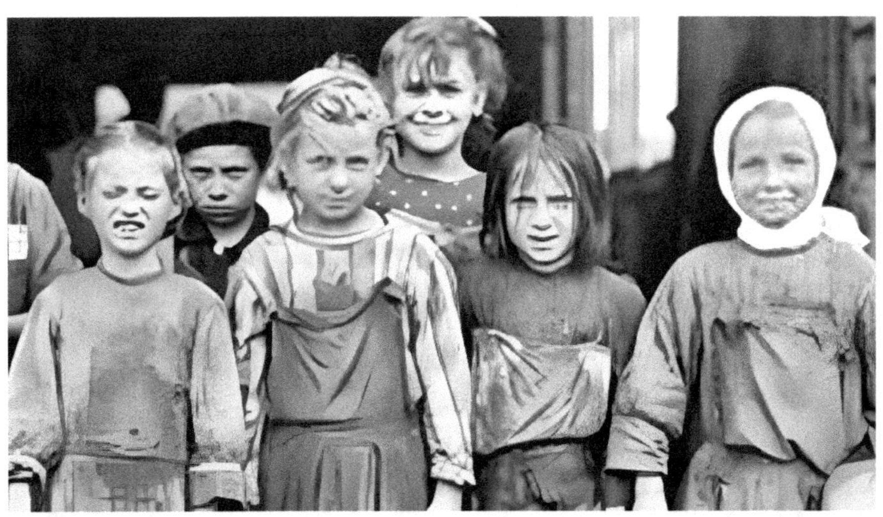

For decades, US citizens have had access to hundreds of varieties of cereals, biscuits, cakes, and other high-carbohydrate and sugary foods. My theory posits that placing a human population in an environment where food is both abundant and inexpensive has led to a form of rapid evolution, resulting in humans becoming more predisposed to converting food into fat and storing it within the body. This gradual evolutionary change has taken approximately six generations to manifest. To reverse this rapid evolution, the US population would need to endure around six generations in a food-deprived environment to resemble a population of similar build and body shape, such as the Russians, who have largely lived in a food-deprived region over a similar period.

I believe that studying the US population over the past 250 years provides the most compelling empirical evidence supporting the thesis that human body shape and size are physiological traits, taking generations to develop and, consequently, generations to reverse. While individuals can make lifestyle changes within their lifetime, they will always be contending with their genetic makeup.

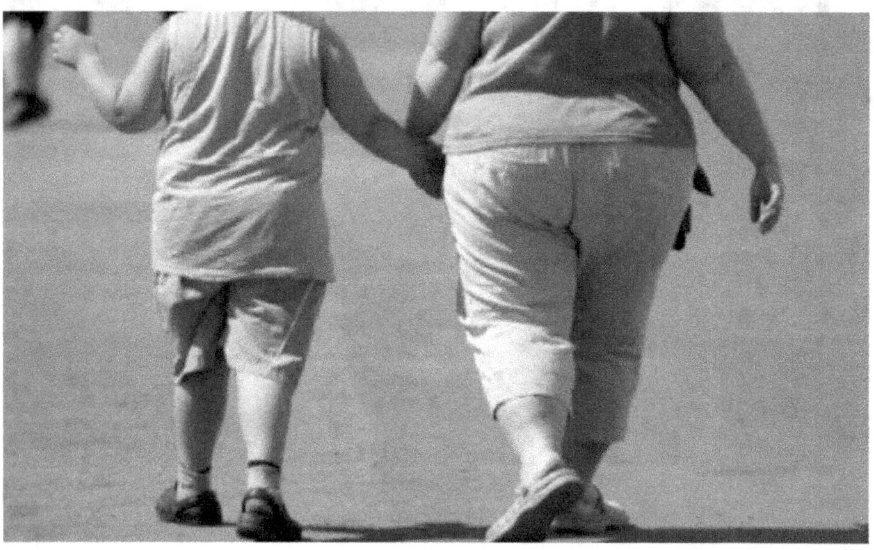

China serves as another compelling example to support my theory. After centuries, if not millennia, of being a food-deprived region, as recently as the 1950's there was widespread famine in China. It also has to be said that as a species we are programmed to eat, whenever on the rare occasions the overabundance of food presents itself. If you image as our species developed it never knew where or when its next meal was going to be available.

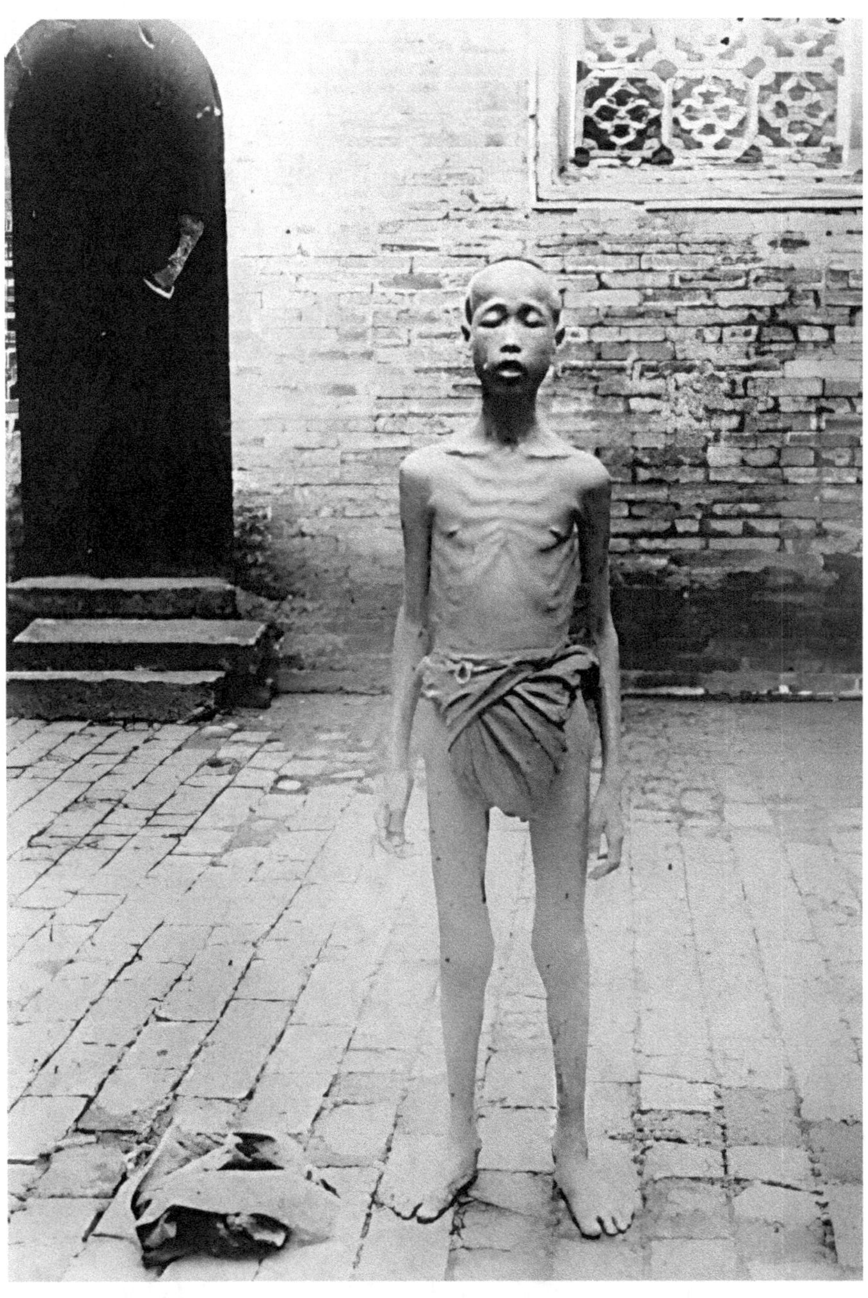

China has undergone significant development over the past three decades. This rapid economic growth has led to an increase in the availability and variety of food, resulting in a rise in obesity among its children for perhaps the first time in its history.

Historically, China faced numerous famines and food shortages, leading to a population that was largely lean and wiry. Generations of scarcity shaped the genetic makeup of the Chinese people, favouring those who could survive on minimal nutrition. However, with the advent of economic reforms in the late 20th century, China experienced unprecedented growth, bringing about dramatic changes in lifestyle and diet.

A study published in The Lancet in 2014 highlighted the alarming rise in childhood obesity in China. It reported that the prevalence of overweight and obesity among children aged 7-18 years increased from 1.1% in 1985 to 17.1% in 2014. This rapid increase correlates with the economic boom that led to greater food availability and the adoption of a more Westernised diet, high in calories, fats, and sugars.

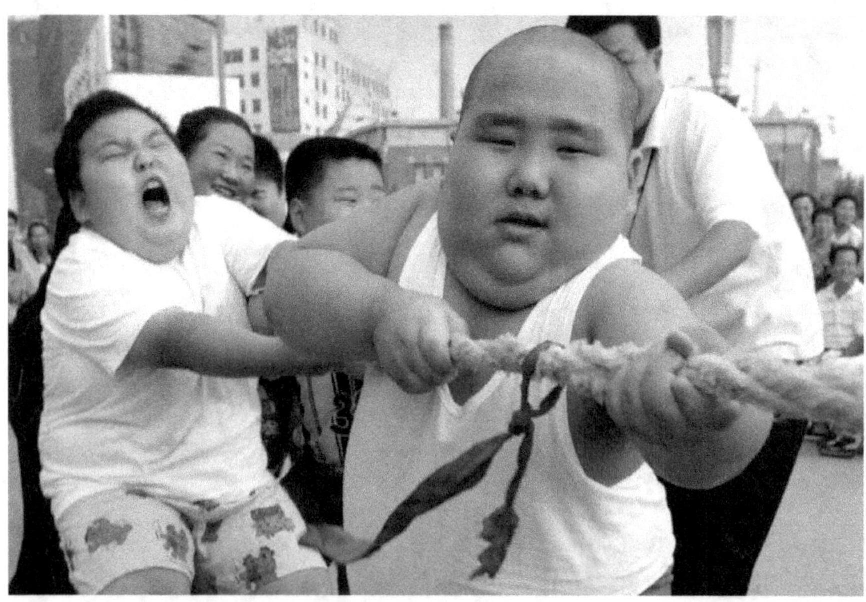

Furthermore, a study by the Chinese Centre for Disease Control and Prevention revealed that urbanisation and the increase in disposable income have significantly altered dietary habits. The traditional Chinese diet, once rich in vegetables and grains, has been supplemented with higher-calorie processed foods and sugary drinks. This shift has been particularly noticeable in urban areas where convenience foods and sedentary lifestyles have become more common.

The rise in obesity in China supports the notion that a population's body size and shape are influenced by generational exposure to environmental factors, such as food availability. As China continues to develop, its population is undergoing a rapid evolutionary change, mirroring the trends observed in the United States. This evidence underscores the argument that while individual lifestyle choices play a role, genetic predisposition shaped by historical and environmental contexts remains a significant factor in determining body size and shape.

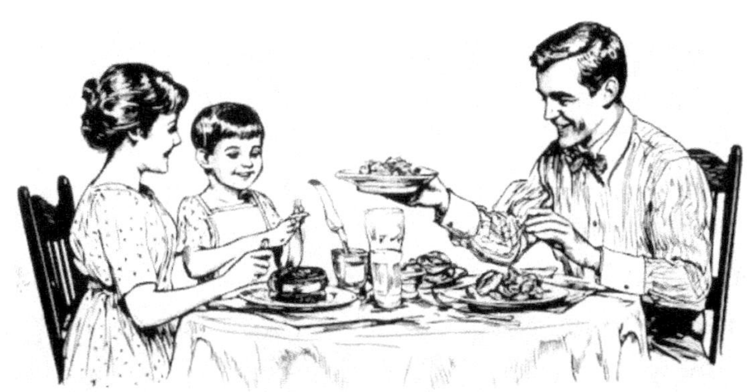

1. Its not all your fault.

Understanding genetic predisposition involves delving into the intricacies of how our genetic makeup influences various traits, including body size, shape, and body mass index (BMI). This concept encompasses the idea that specific genes or genetic variations can predispose individuals to certain physical characteristics, health conditions, or behaviours. However, these predispositions are often influenced by environmental factors and lifestyle choices. The scope of genetic predisposition is broad, covering a wide range of traits and conditions influenced by our genes, from physical attributes like height and weight to more complex traits such as susceptibility to certain diseases or behavioural tendencies.

The historical perspective on genetic studies related to body size and shape reveals a long-standing interest in understanding how genetic factors contribute to these physical attributes. Early studies in genetics, dating back to the early 20th century, began to uncover the role of heredity in determining physical characteristics. Gregor Mendel's pioneering work on inheritance in pea plants laid the groundwork for understanding genetic inheritance, but it wasn't until the advent of modern genetic research tools that scientists could begin to unravel the complex genetic underpinnings of body size and shape. Studies on identical twins, who share the same genetic makeup, have provided valuable insights into the heritability of body size and shape, demonstrating that genetics play a significant role in these traits.

The key genetic factors influencing body size, shape, and BMI are numerous and involve a complex interplay of various genes. Among these, genes involved in growth and development play a crucial role. For example, the human growth hormone (HGH) gene is essential for normal growth and development, affecting height and overall body size. Mutations or variations in this gene can lead to growth disorders, underscoring its importance in determining physical stature. Additionally, the insulin-like growth factor 1 (IGF-1) gene is another critical player in growth regulation. IGF-1 is involved in cell growth and development and has been linked to variations in height and body size among different individuals.

Genes related to metabolism and fat storage are also pivotal in influencing body size, shape, and BMI. The FTO gene, often referred to as the "fat mass and obesity-associated" gene, has garnered significant attention for its association with obesity. Variations in the FTO gene have been linked to increased body weight and a higher propensity for fat storage, making it a key genetic factor in understanding obesity and body composition. Similarly, the leptin gene plays a crucial role in regulating energy balance and body weight. Leptin is a hormone produced by fat cells that signals the brain to regulate food intake and energy expenditure. Variations in the leptin gene can lead to disruptions in this signalling pathway, contributing to obesity and other metabolic disorders.

The role of heritability in body size and composition is substantial, with studies indicating that a significant portion of these traits is inherited from our parents. Heritability estimates for traits like height, weight, and BMI vary, but research suggests that genetic factors account for approximately 60-80% of the variation in these traits. For example, twin studies have shown that identical twins, who share the same genetic makeup, exhibit remarkably similar body sizes and shapes, even when raised in different environments. This high degree of similarity underscores the strong genetic component in determining these physical attributes.

Genetic predisposition also involves exploring the concept of epigenetics, which refers to changes in gene expression that do not involve alterations to the underlying DNA sequence. Epigenetic changes can be influenced by environmental factors, such as diet, stress, and exposure to toxins, and can have lasting effects on an individual's health and physical characteristics. Another example of this might be when we look at the Oceanic or Polynesian people, Polynesian explorers stand among history's most intrepid navigators, their extraordinary voyages across the vast Pacific Ocean leading to the settlement of numerous remote islands.

These brave seafarers, using sophisticated navigational skills honed over generations, embarked on their journeys in outrigger canoes and double-hulled voyaging canoes. The exploration and eventual settlement of these islands, including Hawaii, Easter Island (Rapa Nui), and New Zealand (Aotearoa), began around 1000 CE and extended over several centuries.

The Polynesians hailed from the islands of Tonga, Samoa, and Fiji, and they ventured out into the unknown, guided by the stars, ocean currents, wind patterns, and an intimate understanding of their environment. Their achievements are lionized in the oral traditions and legends passed down through generations. Hawaii was settled around 900-1000 CE, Easter Island around 1200 CE, and New Zealand around 1250-1300 CE. Each of these islands presented its own challenges and opportunities, shaping the cultures that would flourish there.

Polynesian society was structured around a complex system of chiefdoms, with social hierarchies based on lineage and kinship. They were adept farmers and fishermen, cultivating taro, sweet potatoes, and breadfruit, and raising pigs and chickens. Their societies valued art and craftsmanship, as evidenced by their intricate wood carvings, tattoos, and woven textiles. The Polynesians also had a rich spiritual life, with beliefs centred around gods and ancestors, and elaborate rituals and ceremonies to honour them.

The physical and cultural prowess of the Polynesians extended to their remarkable ability to adapt to the harsh and varied environments of the Pacific islands. This adaptability is a testament to their genetic evolution, shaped by the demands of their voyages and the necessity for survival. One critical factor in their adaptation was the need for efficient fat and energy storage, a trait that became hereditary through the process of epigenetics.

As the Polynesians navigated vast oceanic distances, often facing unpredictable weather and scarcity of food, their bodies needed to endure long periods without sustenance. This extreme environment necessitated a physiological adaptation for energy conservation and storage. Over generations, those who could efficiently store fat and convert it into energy during times of scarcity had a survival advantage. Consequently, these traits were passed down, becoming a hallmark of Polynesian genetic makeup.

Epigenetics plays a significant role in this evolutionary process. The environmental pressures of oceanic voyages likely triggered epigenetic changes that enhanced the expression of genes associated with fat storage and energy metabolism. These changes, while not altering the DNA sequence itself, modified how genes were expressed, leading to a body plan optimised for survival in resource-scarce conditions. Such adaptations would have been beneficial not only during voyages but also in the variable environments of newly settled islands.

This epigenetic inheritance ensured that subsequent generations were better equipped to thrive in their challenging surroundings. The capacity for efficient fat storage and energy utilisation became a defining feature of Polynesian physiology, aiding their remarkable colonisation efforts. The interplay between genetic predisposition and environmental demands underscores the dynamic nature of human evolution, illustrating how the Polynesians' legendary voyages left an indelible mark on their genetic legacy.

However just a few hundred years later following the age of discovery, and exposure to western high grain, and high carbohydrate diets what had been a positive trait, resulted in high levels of obesity among, these Oceanic societies

The Dutch famine, known as the "Hongerwinter," was a devastating period in the winter of 1944-1945, during the final year of World War II. As Nazi Germany's grip on the occupied Netherlands weakened, Allied forces advanced, creating a dire situation for the Dutch population. The German blockade, compounded by a harsh winter and deliberate food supply disruptions, resulted in severe food shortages. This famine affected approximately 4.5 million people in the western Netherlands, leading to widespread malnutrition, starvation, and death. The daily caloric intake for adults dropped to as low as 400-800 calories, far below the minimum needed for survival.

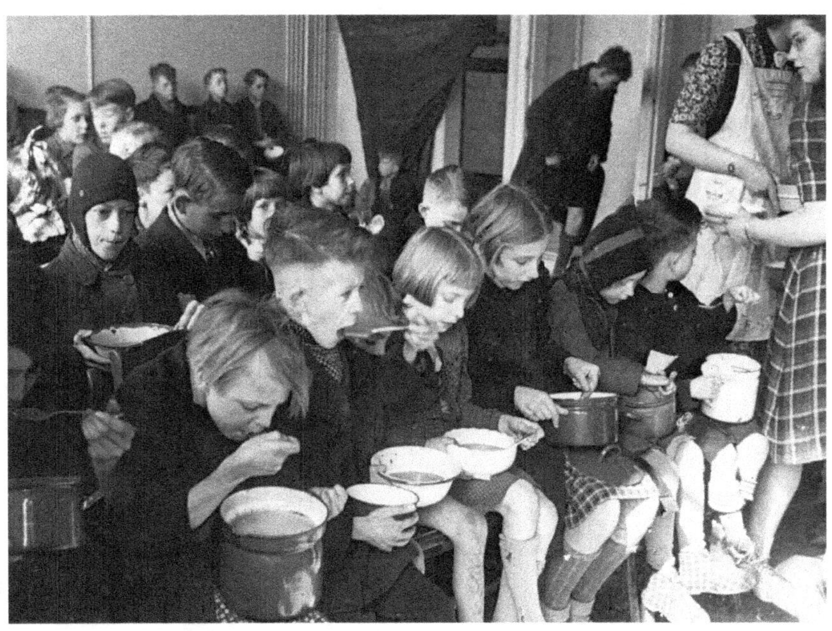

The impact on the population was catastrophic. By the end of the famine, around 22,000 people had died, though some estimates suggest the number could be higher. Those who survived faced severe health issues. Malnutrition led to weakened immune systems, increasing susceptibility to diseases like tuberculosis. Pregnant women were particularly affected, and the famine had profound and lasting effects on the health of their offspring. The long-term consequences included higher rates of chronic conditions such as diabetes, cardiovascular diseases, and mental health disorders among those who were in utero during the famine.

The concept of gene memory, or epigenetic inheritance, provides a framework to understand how such environmental stresses can have enduring effects on subsequent generations. Epigenetics refers to changes in gene expression that do not involve alterations to the underlying DNA sequence. These changes can be induced by various environmental factors, such as nutrition, stress, and toxins. The mechanisms through which epigenetic changes occur include DNA methylation, histone modification, and the action of non-coding RNAs. DNA methylation involves the addition of methyl groups to DNA, typically suppressing gene expression. Histone modifications, such as acetylation or methylation, alter the structure of chromatin, thereby regulating access to DNA and influencing gene activity. Non-coding RNAs can also regulate gene expression by binding to messenger RNAs or modifying chromatin structure.

Studies on the long-term health effects of prenatal exposure to famine have revealed significant insights. Research led by Dr. Tessa Roseboom and her colleagues has been instrumental in uncovering these impacts. They found that individuals who were conceived or in early gestation during the Dutch famine were more likely to suffer from obesity, diabetes, and cardiovascular diseases later in life. This research has demonstrated that prenatal exposure to malnutrition can result in permanent metabolic changes, predisposing individuals to various health conditions.

Dr. Roseboom's findings suggest that the famine altered the epigenetic programming of the unborn children, leading to increased fat storage and altered glucose metabolism as adaptive responses to anticipated food scarcity. These changes, beneficial for survival during famine, become detrimental in an environment with abundant food, contributing to higher rates of metabolic disorders. For instance, the study published in "Molecular and Cellular Endocrinology" in 2001 provided a comprehensive overview of these effects, highlighting how critical periods of development are sensitive to environmental conditions.

Further research, such as the study by Heijmans et al. published in the "Proceedings of the National Academy of Sciences" in 2008, found persistent epigenetic differences in individuals exposed to the famine prenatally. They observed that these individuals had altered DNA methylation patterns in specific genes related to growth and metabolism. This reinforced the idea that early developmental exposures could have lifelong consequences through epigenetic mechanisms.

The broader implications of gene memory extend beyond understanding the impact of the Dutch famine. This concept is crucial for comprehending genetic predispositions to various health conditions and how environmental factors influence gene expression across generations. It challenges the traditional view of genetics as a static blueprint, highlighting the dynamic interplay between genes and the environment. This interplay is evident in the heritability of conditions such as obesity, where both genetic factors and lifestyle contribute to disease risk.

The work of researchers like Dr. Roseboom emphasizes the importance of considering prenatal and early life environments in public health strategies. Understanding epigenetic mechanisms opens new avenues for interventions that could mitigate the long-term health effects of adverse early life experiences. This knowledge is also relevant for addressing health disparities, as populations exposed to different environmental stresses may exhibit distinct epigenetic profiles that influence disease susceptibility.

The Dutch famine provides a stark example of how severe environmental conditions can have lasting effects on human health through epigenetic changes. The research conducted on the survivors of the Hongerwinter has been pivotal in demonstrating the mechanisms of gene memory and its implications for understanding the relationship between genetics and environment. These findings underscore the importance of early life conditions in shaping health outcomes and the potential for epigenetic research to inform public health strategies and interventions aimed at reducing the burden of chronic diseases.

Epigenetics, a term first coined by C.H. Waddington in the 1940s, refers to heritable changes in gene expression that do not involve changes to the underlying DNA sequence. These modifications, which include DNA methylation, histone modification, and non-coding RNA-associated gene silencing, play a crucial role in regulating gene expression. Epigenetics allows for the dynamic regulation of genes in response to environmental cues, enabling organisms to adapt to their surroundings without altering their genetic code. This complex layer of genetic regulation is fundamental in developmental processes and can have profound implications for health and disease.

One of the most fascinating aspects of epigenetics is its sensitivity to environmental factors. Nutrition, stress, exposure to toxins, and lifestyle choices can all influence epigenetic modifications. These factors can lead to changes in gene expression that can have lasting effects on an individual's phenotype. For instance, the diet a person consumes can affect the methylation patterns of genes involved in metabolism and body weight regulation. Similarly, chronic stress can lead to alterations in the expression of genes associated with the stress response, potentially increasing the risk of mental health disorders.

Historical famines provide compelling case studies for understanding the impact of epigenetics and environmental factors on human health. Beyond the well-documented Dutch famine of 1944-1945, other significant events, such as the Great Chinese Famine (1959-1961) and the Siege of Leningrad (1941-1944), offer valuable insights.

The Great Chinese Famine, resulting from a combination of natural disasters and the policy failures of the Great Leap Forward, led to the starvation of millions of people. Research has shown that individuals who were in utero during this period exhibit altered epigenetic markers, which have been linked to increased risks of metabolic disorders, such as type 2 diabetes and obesity, later in life. These epigenetic changes underscore the long-term health impacts of severe nutritional deprivation during critical periods of development.

Similarly, the Siege of Leningrad during World War II, where residents experienced extreme food shortages and malnutrition, has provided important data on the epigenetic consequences of famine. Studies of survivors and their descendants have revealed persistent epigenetic alterations, particularly in genes involved in growth and metabolism. These changes suggest that the environmental stress experienced during the siege had lasting effects on gene expression that could be transmitted to subsequent generations.

The concept of transgenerational epigenetic inheritance further complicates the relationship between genetics and environment. This phenomenon refers to the transmission of epigenetic marks from one generation to the next, potentially affecting the health and development of descendants. For instance, the children and grandchildren of individuals who experienced the Dutch famine have been found to exhibit increased risks of various health issues, including cardiovascular diseases and diabetes, despite not experiencing the famine themselves. This indicates that the epigenetic changes induced by the famine were inherited and continued to influence gene expression in subsequent generations.

The study of transgenerational effects and survival mechanisms highlights the adaptive nature of epigenetic changes. In response to extreme environmental stress, such as famine, the body may undergo epigenetic modifications that enhance survival in resource-scarce environments. These changes can prepare future generations for similar conditions, demonstrating an evolutionary advantage. However, in modern societies where food scarcity is less common, these same epigenetic marks can predispose individuals to obesity and metabolic disorders, illustrating the complex relationship between past and present environments. So in other words it can work both ways the human body will adapt to a famine, will also adapt to a feast, where food is over abundant an adaptation might be to store fat, and slow the body down, it does not matter what your ethnic background it's the environment.

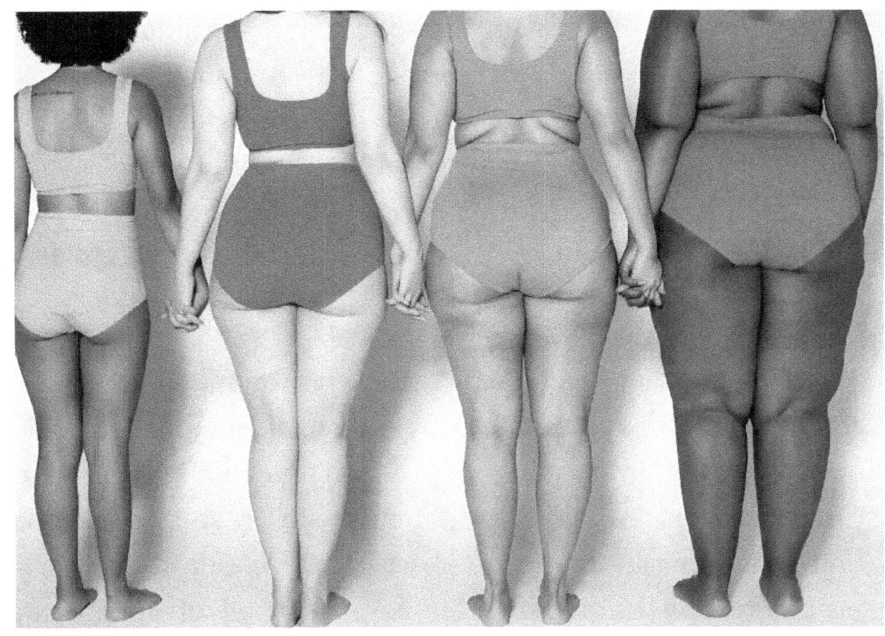

Epigenetics is a dynamic and rapidly evolving field that bridges the gap between genetics and environmental influences. It offers a nuanced understanding of how external factors can shape gene expression and, consequently, health and disease. The impact of nutrition, stress, toxins, and lifestyle choices on epigenetic changes emphasises the importance of considering both genetic and environmental factors in the study of human health. The historical cases of famine illustrate the profound and lasting effects that severe environmental stress can have on epigenetic regulation and health outcomes, not only for those directly affected but also for their descendants.

In examining the role of epigenetics in shaping body size and BMI, it is clear that both genetic predisposition and environmental factors must be taken into account. While genetic factors provide a baseline susceptibility, environmental influences such as diet and lifestyle play a significant role in determining actual outcomes. This understanding has important implications for public health strategies aimed at addressing obesity and metabolic disorders. By recognising the relationship between genes and the environment, interventions can be better tailored to address the underlying causes of these conditions.

The study of epigenetics and environmental influence continues to uncover the intricate mechanisms through which external factors impact gene expression and health. As research progresses, it holds the potential to revolutionise our understanding of heredity, disease prevention, and health promotion. By unravelling the complex web of genetic and environmental interactions, we can develop more effective strategies for improving health outcomes across generations.

The field of epigenetics provides a compelling framework for understanding the intricate relationships between our genes and the environment. Historical events such as the Great Chinese Famine and the Siege of Leningrad illustrate the lasting impact of environmental stress on gene expression and health. The study of transgenerational effects underscores the importance of considering not only immediate environmental influences but also the long-term consequences for future generations. As we continue to explore the complexities of epigenetic regulation, it becomes increasingly clear that both genetic predispositions and environmental factors must be considered in the pursuit of improved health and well-being.

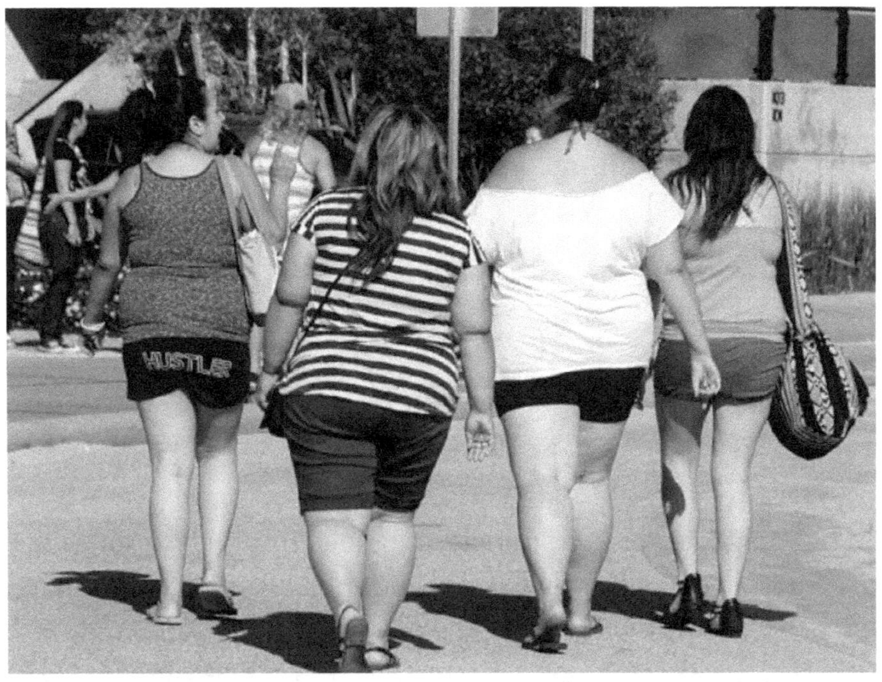

Genetics, by definition, frequently involves the examination of abnormalities. This suggests that it is feasible to describe what is normal; but, because this is so difficult, researchers prefer to examine individuals in terms of variety rather than comparing them to an abstract "norm." One of the most widespread myths about our genes is that they control all human qualities, which can lead to prejudice against people with specific gene combinations or genotypes. A single genetic mutation may occasionally predict a human trait. However, in most circumstances, an individual is a unique, complicated result of several interactions between genes, prenatal conditions, the environment, and lifestyle.

2. Rapid Evolution

Island biogeography, a subfield of biogeography, examines the distribution of species on islands and their unique evolutionary adaptations. The isolation of islands creates natural laboratories where species undergo rapid evolutionary changes. These changes are often driven by the need to adapt to limited resources, lack of predators, and other unique environmental conditions, leading to phenomena such as island dwarfism, where species evolve to a smaller size, and gigantism, where species evolve to a larger size. This chapter explores these evolutionary processes, providing insights into the mechanisms and examples that illustrate the dynamic nature of evolution in isolated environments.

Island dwarfism, also known as insular dwarfism, is a fascinating process of rapid evolutionary change where large species evolve into smaller forms when isolated on islands. This phenomenon is particularly evident in mammals, reptiles, and birds. The factors driving island dwarfism include limited resources, which necessitate smaller body sizes for efficient energy use, and the absence of predators, which reduces the need for larger sizes as a defence mechanism. A notable example is the Sicilian dwarf elephant (Palaeoloxodon falconeri) and the Cyprus dwarf elephant (Palaeoloxodon cypriotes), illustrating how these majestic creatures evolved into significantly smaller forms due to the constraints and pressures of island life.

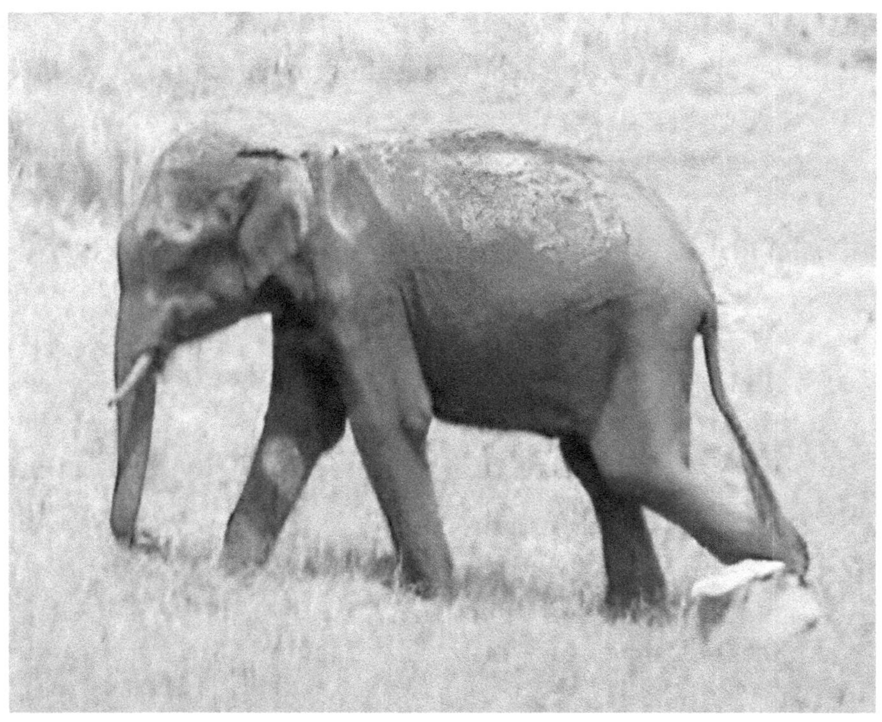

The Sicilian dwarf elephant, Palaeoloxodon falconeri, lived approximately 800,000 to 10,000 years ago on the Mediterranean island of Sicily. Evolved from larger mainland relatives, adults stood around one metre tall at the shoulder. The island's limited food supply and the absence of large predators drove this size reduction. Similarly, the Cyprus dwarf elephant, Palaeoloxodon cypriotes, existed on the island of Cyprus during the late Pleistocene epoch, with adults just over a metre tall. The evolutionary pressures on Cyprus mirrored those on Sicily, leading to similar dwarfing in the elephant population.

Other examples of rapid evolutionary changes in island species include the Channel Island fox (Urocyon littoralis) and flightless birds such as the flightless cormorant of the Galápagos Islands. The Channel Island fox, found on the Channel Islands off the coast of California, is a striking case of rapid evolution. Descended from the mainland grey fox, these foxes evolved into a smaller, distinct species in a relatively short period, adapting to the unique conditions of their island habitats. The absence of large predators and the limited availability of resources drove this species to become smaller and more specialised in its diet and behaviour.

Flightless birds provide another compelling example of rapid evolutionary changes on islands. The flightless cormorant of the Galápagos Islands has evolved to lose its ability to fly, a trait that is energy-intensive and unnecessary in an environment without terrestrial predators. Instead, these birds have developed enhanced diving abilities to exploit the rich marine resources surrounding their island home. This adaptation highlights the remarkable flexibility of evolutionary processes in response to isolated environments.

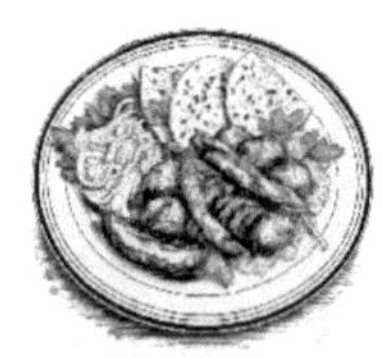

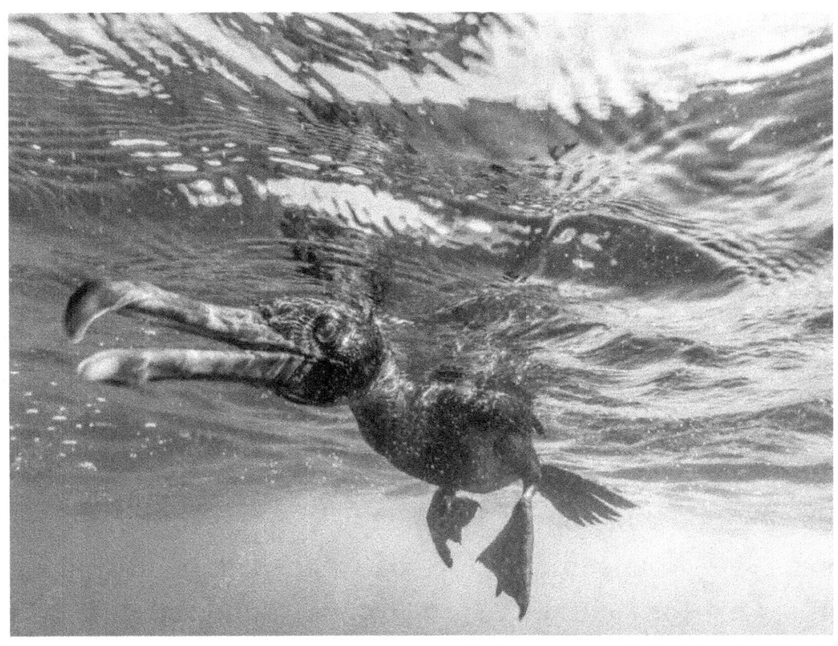

A comparison between island dwarfism and gigantism reveals intriguing insights into the varied responses of species to island isolation. While some species evolve to become smaller, others undergo gigantism, becoming significantly larger than their mainland relatives. The Komodo dragon (Varanus komodoensis) is a prime example of island gigantism. Found on the Indonesian islands of Komodo, Rinca, Flores, and Gili Motang, the Komodo dragon is the largest living species of lizard, growing up to three metres in length. The absence of large mammalian predators and the availability of large prey, such as deer, drove the Komodo dragon to evolve into a giant predator, illustrating how different evolutionary pressures can lead to vastly different outcomes in isolated environments.

Island biogeography offers a unique lens through which to study evolutionary processes, as the isolation provided by islands accelerates changes that might take much longer on the mainland. The case studies of the Sicilian and Cyprus dwarf elephants demonstrate how significant evolutionary changes can occur in relatively short geological timescales when species are subjected to the pressures of limited resources and lack of predators. Similarly, the examples of the Channel Island fox and flightless birds underscore the adaptive flexibility of species in response to island environments.

The study of rapid evolutionary changes in isolated species enhances our understanding of evolutionary mechanisms and provides valuable insights into the broader principles of adaptation and survival. These insights have implications for conservation biology, highlighting the importance of preserving isolated environments where unique evolutionary processes can unfold. Furthermore, understanding these mechanisms can inform efforts to manage and protect species threatened by habitat fragmentation and other human-induced changes to their environments.

The study of island biogeography and evolutionary adaptations reveals the dynamic and often rapid nature of evolutionary change in isolated species. Island dwarfism, exemplified by the Sicilian and Cyprus dwarf elephants, showcases how species can evolve smaller sizes in response to limited resources and predator-free environments. Similarly, other rapid evolutionary changes, such as those seen in the Channel Island fox and flightless birds, highlight the adaptive flexibility of species. The comparison between island dwarfism and gigantism, with the Komodo dragon as a prominent example of the latter, further underscores the diverse outcomes of evolutionary processes in isolated environments. These studies deepen our understanding of evolution and underscore the importance of conserving unique habitats where such processes can continue to unfold.

The synthesis of gene memory and epigenetics with the concept of genetic predisposition has revolutionised our understanding of human development, particularly in relation to body size and shape. Gene memory refers to the biological inheritance of experiences and environmental factors that affect gene expression. Epigenetics involves changes in organisms caused by modification of gene expression rather than alteration of the genetic code itself. Together, these fields provide a compelling framework for exploring how our genes and environment interact to shape our physical attributes.

Genetic predisposition has long been understood as the innate potential coded in our DNA, influencing traits such as height, body composition, and susceptibility to certain diseases. This genetic blueprint does not operate in isolation. Early-life environmental conditions can significantly influence genetic expression, leading to variations in body size and shape among individuals with similar genetic backgrounds. For instance, prenatal exposure to stressors, nutrition, and other external factors can leave lasting marks on the genome, affecting an individual's growth trajectory and metabolic pathways.

The study of human genetics is significantly different from how biologists research other living forms. Although human experimentation is generally prohibited in our culture, the practice of medicine has offered a more complete picture of our species' anatomy and physiology than any other organism on the planet. Vast amounts of observational data incorporated in patient medical records provide insights into normal human variation while also documenting the causes and progression of various disorders. Medical research in human genetics is currently yielding clinical advances that are a revolution. It promises to address fundamental issues about our human nature, explain disorders, and lead to efficient treatments. Understanding the genetics of human life is so immediately applicable to each of us as individuals..

The balance between genetic predisposition and environmental influence can be encapsulated in the 70% genetic versus 30% diet and lifestyle model. This model suggests that while a significant portion of human body size, shape, and body fat mass index is predetermined by genetic factors, environmental conditions and lifestyle choices also play a crucial role. This balance is dynamic and can shift depending on various factors, including the timing and intensity of environmental exposures.

For instance, the work of Weaver et al. (2004) on maternal behaviour in rats has shown that early-life environmental conditions, such as maternal care, can lead to epigenetic changes that influence stress responses and metabolic health. These findings suggest that nurturing environments can mitigate some of the negative effects of genetic predisposition, highlighting the importance of supportive and healthy early-life conditions. Conversely, adverse environments can exacerbate genetic vulnerabilities, leading to poorer health outcomes.

In public health and disease prevention, understanding the connection between genetic predisposition and environmental influences is paramount. By recognising that early-life conditions can have a lasting impact on gene expression and health, we can develop more effective interventions and policies aimed at improving health outcomes. For example, public health initiatives that ensure adequate nutrition for pregnant women and young children can help mitigate the effects of adverse prenatal exposures, reducing the risk of obesity and related diseases in later life.

Furthermore, insights from epigenetics can inform personalised medicine approaches. By considering an individual's genetic predisposition and environmental history, healthcare providers can tailor prevention and treatment strategies to better address specific health risks. This personalised approach can lead to more effective management of conditions such as obesity, diabetes, and cardiovascular diseases, which are influenced by both genetic and environmental factors.

Real-world implications of this integrated perspective extend beyond individual health to broader societal outcomes. For instance, policies aimed at reducing environmental toxins, improving access to healthy foods, and promoting physical activity can have a significant impact on public health. By creating environments that support healthy genetic expression, we can improve population health and reduce the burden of chronic diseases.

The study of gene memory, epigenetics, and their interaction with genetic predisposition provides a nuanced understanding of human development. These understanding challenges the deterministic view of genetics, highlighting the plasticity of gene expression in response to environmental conditions. It also underscores the importance of early-life interventions in shaping long-term health outcomes.

The integration of gene memory and epigenetics with the concept of genetic predisposition offers a comprehensive framework for understanding human body size and shape.

Early-life environmental conditions play a crucial role in shaping genetic expression, and the balance between genetic predisposition and environmental influence is dynamic. Real-world implications of this knowledge include the potential for targeted public health interventions and personalised medicine approaches that can improve health outcomes and reduce the prevalence of chronic diseases. This integrated perspective highlights the importance of considering both genetic and environmental factors in the quest to understand and enhance human health.

The dynamic dependence between genetics and environment is a subject of immense fascination and complexity. This relationship is not merely a one-way street where genetics determines every aspect of our being, but rather a multifaceted interaction where environment and lifestyle can significantly alter genetic predispositions. This intricate dance between our DNA and the world around us shapes not only our physical attributes such as body size and health but also our susceptibility to various diseases and conditions.

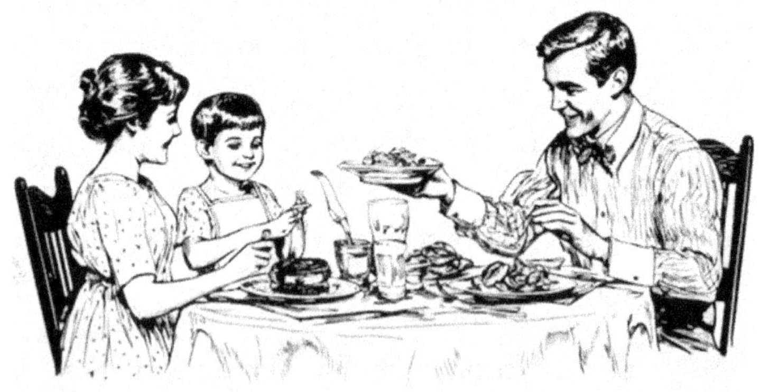

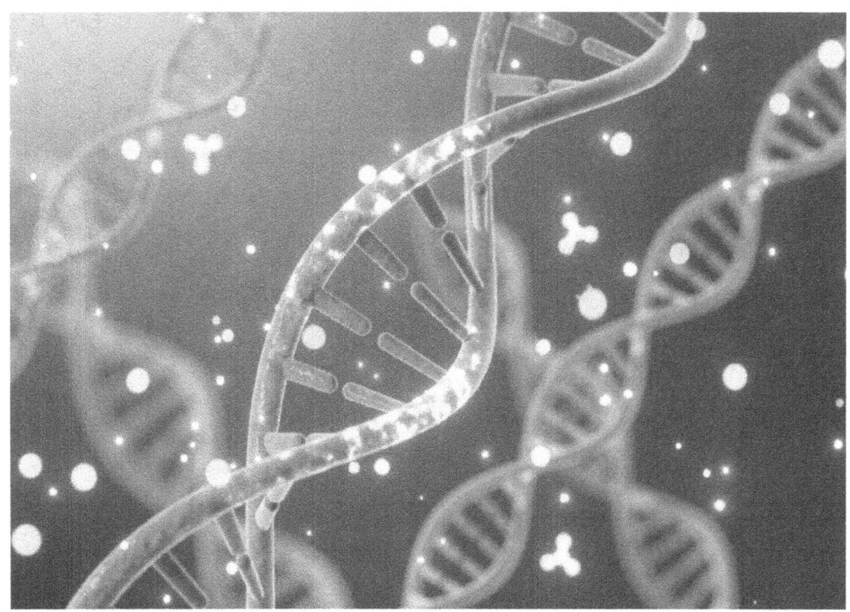

To truly appreciate the extent of this relationship, we must delve into the concept of epigenetics, which offers a window into how environmental factors can modify genetic expression. Epigenetics refers to heritable changes in gene function that do not involve changes in the DNA sequence itself. These changes can be triggered by various environmental factors including diet, stress, and exposure to toxins. One of the most striking examples of epigenetic influence is observed in the studies of prenatal exposure to famine. Research conducted by Roseboom et al. (2001) and Heijmans et al. (2008) provides compelling evidence of how severe nutritional deprivation during critical periods of development can lead to persistent epigenetic changes that affect health outcomes in later life.

The Dutch Hunger Winter of 1944-1945 serves as a poignant case study. During this period, a severe famine struck the Netherlands due to a German blockade, leading to extreme malnutrition among the population. Studies on individuals who were in utero during this famine have shown that they have higher incidences of metabolic diseases such as obesity and type 2 diabetes in adulthood. This phenomenon is believed to result from epigenetic modifications that occurred during fetal development, programming the body to store fat more efficiently as a survival mechanism in response to anticipated scarcity.

Another illustrative case is the impact of maternal behaviour on the epigenetic programming of offspring. Weaver et al. (2004) demonstrated in their study on rats that the quality of maternal care, particularly the frequency of licking and grooming, could alter the epigenetic state of genes involved in stress responses in the offspring. Pups that received high levels of maternal care exhibited lower levels of stress hormones and were more resilient to stress in later life, compared to those that received less maternal care. This research underscores the profound influence of early environmental factors on genetic expression and long-term health outcomes.

The study of body size and health further exemplifies the necessity of a holistic approach. While genetics play a significant role in determining body size, the environment in which an individual lives can either amplify or mitigate these genetic predispositions. The "thrifty gene" hypothesis proposed by James Neel in 1962 suggests that certain populations have genetic adaptations that enable them to store fat more efficiently, an advantage in times of food scarcity. However, in modern environments where high-calorie foods are abundant, these same genetic traits predispose individuals to obesity and related health issues.

O'Rahilly and Farooqi (2008) discuss how obesity, a condition with a strong genetic component, is highly sensitive to environmental influences. They point out that while certain genetic mutations can predispose individuals to obesity, the expression of these genes can be significantly affected by factors such as diet, physical activity, and even social and economic status. For instance, individuals with a genetic predisposition to obesity may never develop the condition if they maintain a healthy lifestyle, indicating the crucial role of the environment in shaping health outcomes.

The island rule, a principle in evolutionary biology, provides another intriguing example of the interaction between genetics and environment. According to this rule, small animals tend to evolve into larger forms on islands, while large animals tend to become smaller. This phenomenon is driven by the unique environmental pressures of island habitats, such as limited resources and the absence of certain predators. Lomolino (2005) and Van der Knaap (1996) document cases like the dwarf elephants of Sicily and the gigantism observed in certain rodent species, demonstrating how isolation and environmental constraints can lead to rapid evolutionary changes in body size.

Moreover, the influence of environment on genetic expression is evident in the study of rapid evolutionary changes in both humans and animals. Hewlett and Lamb (2005) highlight how hunter-gatherer societies, which represent the majority of human evolutionary history, adapted their physical and behavioural traits to their specific environments. These adaptations are not just a product of genetic selection but also of cultural practices and environmental interactions that influence genetic expression over generations.

A holistic understanding of body size and health requires integrating knowledge from genetics, epigenetics, nutrition, and environmental science. While genetics provides the blueprint, the environment can modify, enhance, or suppress the expression of these genetic instructions. For example, a person may have a genetic predisposition for a larger body size, but environmental factors such as diet, exercise, and stress levels will determine whether this potential is realised. This interaction suggests that addressing health issues like obesity requires more than just understanding genetic risk; it necessitates considering the broader environmental and lifestyle factors that influence gene expression.

A doughnut-shaped red blood cell and a neurone in the brain appear so unlike that it is difficult to realise they are from the same organism or even species. However, both sorts of cells are the result of a single "recipe book." They share the same genome but use it in distinct ways as they grow and develop. The same collection of data generates hundreds of different sorts of cells with various appearances and behaviours. When an egg is fertilised, it reproduces and differentiates into around 100 trillion cells that work together to become a human being. Genetics originated as a study of hereditary patterns, often in adult plants and animals. That is still the goal of population genetics, which analyses how a group's genes vary from generation to generation, and hereditary patterns are critical in the search for genes linked to disease. However, as scientists have learnt more about what genes are made of and how they function, their attention has altered slightly.

Until the second half of the nineteenth century, people only had a basic understanding of heredity. The ancient Jews noted that haemophilia, a fatal condition in which the blood fails to coagulate, ran in families and could be passed down from mother to son. While every newborn boy had to be circumcised, an exemption may be granted if the disease ran in his mother's family. Farmers and breeders were aware that gathering the seeds of plants with particular traits or permitting select animals to marry may alter crops and animals. However, until the late nineteenth century, knowledge of how creatures transmitted features on to their offspring was sparse.

Today, scientists believe that a human cell encodes between 20,000 and 25,000 genes, which is around three times the number found in a yeast cell and less than twice the number found in a fly. These data were only available in the early years of the twenty-first century, when scientists had learnt a lot about the chemistry and functions of genes and got whole genome sequences from creatures. Yet, a century ago, even before knowing that genes were made of DNA, Thomas Hunt Morgan's laboratory made incredible progress in finding novel genes and characterising their properties and activities. Morgan and his colleagues' results have had a significant impact on the advancement of human genetics, setting the framework for the discovery of new genes and mutations associated with disease.

In public health, strategies that incorporate genetic predisposition are increasingly important. Personalised medicine is at the forefront of this approach, utilising genetic information to tailor medical treatments to individual patients. This can lead to more effective and targeted therapies, reducing the trial-and-error approach of traditional treatments. Personalised medicine can identify the most effective medications with the fewest side effects based on an individual's genetic makeup, significantly improving patient outcomes. Moreover, understanding genetic predisposition can inform nutritional and lifestyle interventions, allowing for personalised recommendations that can prevent or manage diseases. For example, individuals with a genetic risk for high cholesterol can receive specific dietary guidelines to manage their condition proactively.

Looking ahead, the future of research in this field promises exciting breakthroughs. Advances in genome sequencing technologies and bioinformatics are enabling more precise identification of genetic variants associated with diseases. This knowledge can lead to the development of novel therapies that target specific genetic mutations. Additionally, research into gene editing technologies, such as CRISPR-Cas9, holds the potential to correct genetic defects at the source, offering the possibility of curing genetic diseases. Furthermore, the study of epigenetics is opening new avenues for understanding how environmental factors influence gene expression, leading to innovative strategies for disease prevention and management. As our understanding of the genetic basis of health and disease continues to expand, so too will our ability to develop personalised, effective interventions.

Building a human body necessitates the development of hundreds of distinct types of cells with vastly varying looks and behaviours. They all come from a single cell and have the same genome. Despite this, they develop distinct properties since each type of cell has a unique set of genes. A typical human cell may only use one-third or four of its genes. That set dictates the proteins it contains, its form, and the stimuli it may respond to. By appreciating this intricate relationship, we can better understand human development and health, paving the way for more effective and personalised approaches to healthcare and disease prevention.

3. Environmental Influences

The rapid pace of evolutionary changes has provided significant insights into conservation and biodiversity, offering critical lessons for the protection of endangered species and human health. Understanding these dynamic processes, especially through the lens of island biogeography, evolutionary adaptations, and maintaining biodiversity in changing environments, can greatly enhance our strategies and public health initiatives.

Island biogeography, as articulated by Robert MacArthur and E.O. Wilson in the 1960s, emphasises the unique evolutionary pressures faced by species on islands. These environments serve as natural laboratories for studying rapid evolutionary changes due to their isolation and relatively simplified ecosystems. Notable examples include the dwarf elephants of Sicily, such as Palaeoloxodon falconeri, which evolved smaller sizes due to limited resources and the absence of large predators. This phenomenon, known as the "island rule," illustrates how species undergo significant morphological changes in response to their environment.

Lessons from island biogeography can be directly applied to modern conservation efforts. For instance, the rapid adaptation of other species to isolated environments can help us better understand our own heterogeneity and connectivity. Creating wildlife corridors and protected areas that mimic the isolation of islands can foster similar evolutionary processes, promoting the resilience and adaptability of species. Additionally, understanding these evolutionary mechanisms can help in designing more effective captive breeding programmes by considering the environmental conditions that drive adaptive changes.

Maintaining biodiversity in changing environments is essential for the overall health and stability of ecosystems. Biodiversity acts as a buffer against environmental fluctuations, enhancing the resilience of ecosystems to disturbances such as climate change, habitat loss, and invasive species. Rapid evolutionary changes contribute to this resilience by fostering genetic diversity and adaptive potential within populations. As seen in the case of island species, evolutionary pressures can lead to the development of unique traits that enable species to exploit new niches and resources.

A human embryo begins as a fertilised egg that is totipotent, meaning it can develop into any cell type in the body. It multiplies and creates totipotent embryonic stem cells. However, as the embryo reaches the size of 32 cells, it begins to specialise swiftly. One reason for this is that the giant egg cell duplicates its nucleus and subdivides for a while without growing larger; the newborn cells emerge in parts of the original cell that are not identical. Epigenetic research, such as the work by Weaver et al. (2004), has shown that maternal behaviour can induce lasting changes in the stress response of offspring, highlighting the interplay between environment and genetics.

These findings suggest that public health interventions should consider the long-term effects of early-life environmental conditions on health outcomes. For instance, improving maternal nutrition and reducing prenatal stress can have far-reaching benefits for the health of future generations. Additionally, understanding the epigenetic mechanisms underlying rapid evolutionary changes can inform the development of personalised medicine approaches, tailoring interventions based on an individual's genetic and epigenetic profile.

Emerging research on gene-environment interactions, particularly in the context of rapid evolutionary changes, provides a framework for developing holistic health strategies. By examining the genetic and epigenetic responses to environmental pressures, scientists can identify critical windows for intervention and develop targeted therapies that mitigate the risk of disease. This approach is particularly relevant in the face of global environmental changes, which pose new challenges to both human health and biodiversity.

The insights gained from studying rapid evolutionary changes offer valuable lessons human health and disease prevention. The principles of island biogeography highlight the importance of habitat heterogeneity and connectivity in promoting adaptive responses. Understanding the evolutionary adaptations that confer resilience can guide targeted interventions to protect endangered species and maintain biodiversity in changing environments. Moreover, the application of epigenetic research to public health underscores the significance of early-life conditions and gene-environment interactions in shaping health outcomes. By integrating these insights into public health strategies, we can enhance the resilience of human populations in the face of ongoing environmental challenges.

The history of the United States is profoundly intertwined with the waves of migration that have continually reshaped its demographic landscape. Over the past 250 years, the U.S. has evolved from a nascent collection of colonies into a global superpower, largely fuelled by the influx of diverse populations seeking better opportunities. This narrative examines the historical context of U.S. population migration, with a specific focus on immigrants from famine-stricken regions such as Ireland and other European countries. It explores the initial conditions these populations faced in their homelands, the challenges they encountered upon arrival, and how they adapted to an environment characterised by an abundance of resources, significantly altering their genetic and physical makeup over generations.

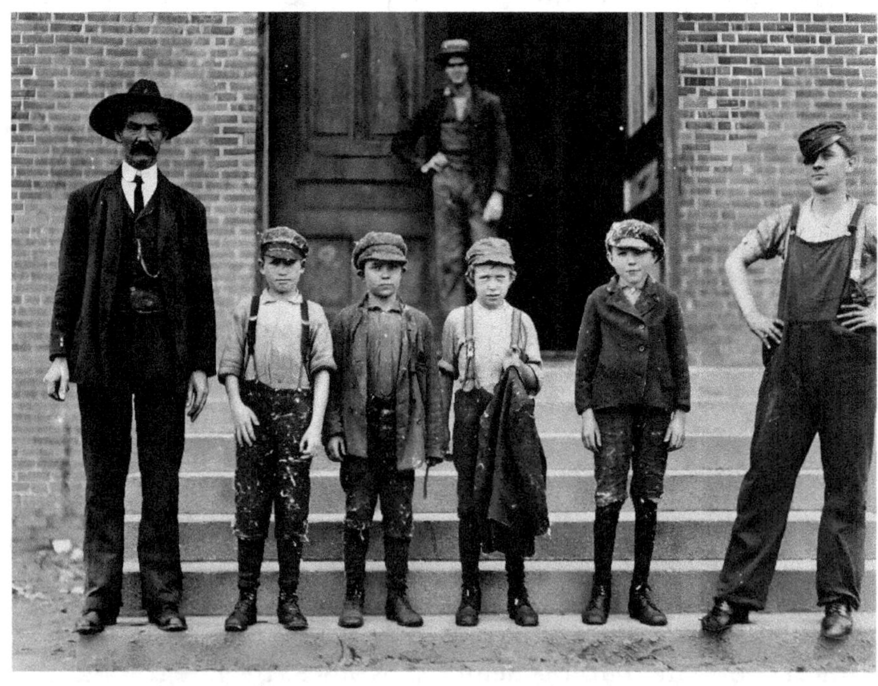

The story of U.S. immigration is marked by distinct waves, each bringing a unique set of people whose lives were irrevocably altered by their decision to migrate. The late 18th and early 19th centuries saw the first significant wave of European immigrants, primarily from Britain, Germany, and the Netherlands. These early settlers were escaping various hardships, including religious persecution, economic instability, and political unrest. The American promise of freedom and land ownership attracted many who were eager to start anew.

The mid-19th century brought a dramatic shift with the arrival of the Irish. The Great Famine of 1845-1852, caused by a potato blight, devastated Ireland, leading to mass starvation and disease. Approximately one million people died, and another million fled, with many finding refuge in the United States. The Irish immigrants arrived in desperate conditions, often malnourished and weakened by the arduous journey. They settled in urban centres like New York, Boston, and Philadelphia, where they faced severe discrimination and were relegated to the most menial jobs. However, over time, they became integral to the labour force, particularly in the construction of infrastructure such as railroads and canals.

Parallel to the Irish influx was the migration of Germans, who, fleeing the political turmoil and economic hardship of the 1848 revolutions, brought with them skills and trades that contributed to America's industrial growth. Unlike the Irish, many Germans settled in rural areas, particularly in the Midwest, where they established farming communities that thrived and expanded.

As the 19th century progressed, other European groups followed. Italians, fleeing economic deprivation and political instability, arrived in large numbers in the late 19th and early

20th centuries. They settled primarily in northeastern cities, forming tight-knit communities that maintained cultural traditions while gradually assimilating into American society. Eastern European Jews, escaping pogroms and persecution, also arrived during this period, contributing significantly to the cultural and economic fabric of cities like New York.

The environmental conditions in the immigrants' home countries were often harsh and unforgiving. In Ireland, the reliance on a single crop, the potato, made the population exceptionally vulnerable to disease and famine. The potato blight that caused the Great Famine was a catastrophe of unparalleled magnitude, decimating the population and forcing survivors to seek refuge abroad. Similarly, in Italy, the combination of poor agricultural conditions, high taxes, and overpopulation created a dire situation that compelled many to emigrate.

Upon arriving in the United States, these immigrant populations encountered an environment vastly different from their homelands. The abundance of food and resources contrasted sharply with the scarcity they had left behind. This sudden change in diet and living conditions had profound effects on their health and physical development. Initially, many immigrants suffered from malnutrition and diseases related to their impoverished conditions. However, the availability of diverse and plentiful food sources eventually led to improvements in their overall health and well-being.

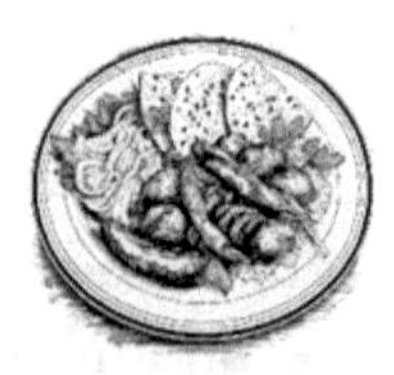

Adaptation to the new environment was not merely a matter of survival but also involved significant changes in lifestyle and diet. Immigrants who had once subsisted on limited and nutritionally deficient diets in their homelands now had access to a variety of foods rich in protein and other essential nutrients. This dietary shift contributed to better physical development in subsequent generations. For instance, children of Irish and Italian immigrants, born and raised in the U.S., often exhibited greater height and better health than their parents, reflecting the impact of improved nutrition and living conditions.

The genetic response to these new environmental conditions is a critical aspect of this narrative. Over generations, the descendants of these immigrants exhibited changes that can be understood through the lens of epigenetics. Studies, such as those conducted by Roseboom et al. (2001) and Heijmans et al. (2008), have shown that environmental factors, including nutrition, can lead to persistent epigenetic changes that affect gene expression and can be inherited by subsequent generations. This concept helps explain how populations that once suffered from famine-related malnutrition adapted to environments with abundant food supplies, resulting in observable changes in physical traits and health outcomes.

The phenomenon of rapid adaptation is also evident in the changing body composition of the U.S. population. The initial immigrants, who arrived undernourished and often in poor health, gave rise to generations that benefited from the availability of nutritious food and better living conditions. This transition can be partly attributed to the genetic and epigenetic changes that occurred as these populations adjusted to their new environment.

By the mid-20th century, the U.S. had become a melting pot of ethnicities, each contributing to the nation's growth and development. The prosperity of the post-World War II era further accelerated changes in lifestyle and diet. The rise of the middle class, suburban living, and the proliferation of processed foods marked a significant shift in American dietary habits. These changes, coupled with a more sedentary lifestyle, have contributed to the current obesity epidemic in the U.S.

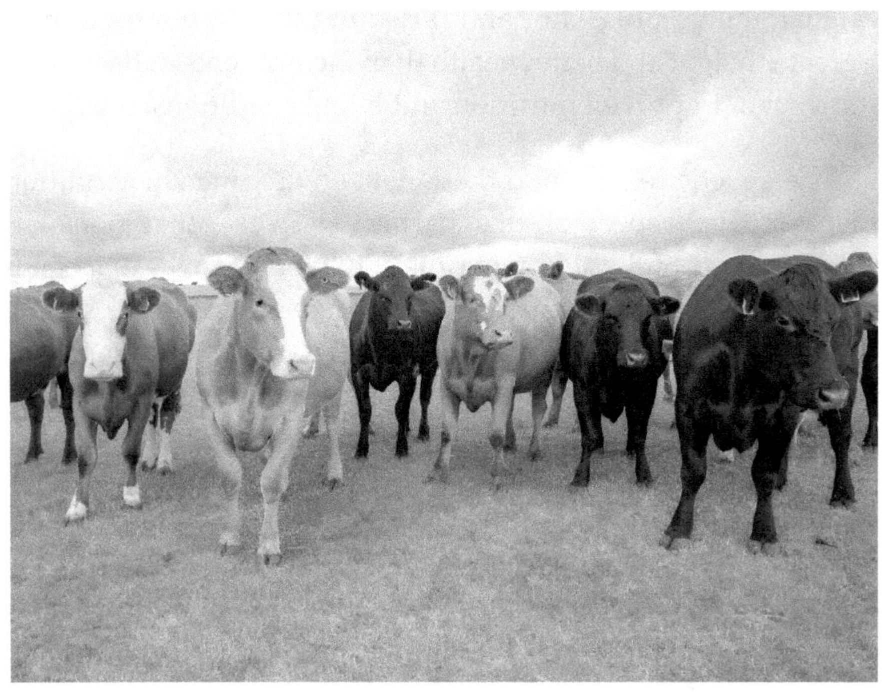

The concept that a significant portion of human body size, shape, and body fat mass index is predetermined by genetic factors is supported by the study of gene memory and epigenetics. The rapid evolution of the U.S. population from famine-ridden immigrants to one of the most obese populations globally is a testament to the interconnected relationship between genetics and environmental factors. As O'Rahilly and Farooqi (2008) have noted, human obesity is a heritable neuro-behavioural disorder highly sensitive to environmental conditions. The abundance of food and changes in dietary habits over generations have played a crucial role in this transformation.

The transformation of immigrant populations in the U.S. highlights the significant impact of environmental conditions on genetic and physical development. The initial body composition of these populations, shaped by the harsh conditions in their homelands, underwent profound changes as they adapted to the abundance of resources in the U.S. This adaptation process, influenced by both genetic and epigenetic factors, underscores the inescapable fact that there is a connection between heredity and environment in shaping human health and physical traits.

The historical context of U.S. population migration reveals a complex narrative of adaptation and transformation. Immigrants from famine-ridden countries like Ireland and other parts of Europe arrived in desperate conditions, only to find themselves in a land of abundance. This drastic change in environment triggered significant genetic and epigenetic responses, leading to observable changes in physical development and health over generations. The evolution of the U.S. population, from malnourished immigrants to a nation grappling with obesity, exemplifies the profound impact of environmental factors on human biology. The study of this transformation provides valuable insights into the ongoing research of genetics and environment, offering a deeper understanding of how populations adapt and evolve in response to changing conditions.

Mutations are frequently shown as odd events that provide humans superhuman abilities or transform people into monsters in science fiction books and films such as the X-Men series and the Heroes television series. In actuality, all humans are born with mutations that result in individual genomes (save for identical twins, whose genes are identical). While many mutations have no discernible effect or have minor effects on cell chemistry, others may affect the entire body by altering how cells behave and organs develop. They may cause sickness or abnormalities.

The understanding of genetic factors influencing body composition has evolved significantly over the years. Initially, the focus was primarily on single gene mutations that resulted in dramatic effects on body weight and fat distribution. For example, mutations in the leptin gene, which plays a crucial role in regulating energy balance and body weight, were found to cause severe obesity. Leptin deficiency disrupts the feedback mechanism that signals satiety to the brain, leading to excessive food intake and weight gain.

However, the genetic architecture of body composition is far more complex, involving numerous genes that each contribute small effects. Genome-wide association studies (GWAS) have identified hundreds of loci associated with body mass index (BMI), a commonly used measure of body composition. These loci include genes involved in lipid metabolism, insulin signalling, and adipogenesis, reflecting the multifactorial nature of obesity and body fat distribution. For instance, the FTO gene is one of the most robustly associated with obesity, influencing food intake and energy expenditure. Individuals with certain variants of the FTO gene are more likely to have higher BMIs and increased body fat.

Scientific studies provide robust evidence supporting the genetic predisposition to obesity and other body composition traits. Twin studies, which compare the similarities in BMI between monozygotic (identical) twins and dizygotic (fraternal) twins, have been instrumental in estimating the heritability of these traits. Heritability estimates for BMI typically range from 40% to 70%, underscoring the significant genetic contribution. Furthermore, adoption studies, where the BMI of adopted children is compared to that of their biological and adoptive parents, reinforce the genetic influence. These studies consistently show a stronger correlation with biological parents, even when the children are raised in different environments.

The role of epigenetics has also garnered attention in understanding the genetic basis for body composition. Epigenetic modifications, such as DNA methylation and histone modification, can influence gene expression without altering the underlying DNA sequence. Environmental factors, including diet, stress, and prenatal nutrition, can induce epigenetic changes that affect body composition. The Dutch Famine of 1944-1945, for example, provided a unique natural experiment to study the long-term effects of prenatal exposure to starvation. Individuals exposed to the famine in utero exhibited increased susceptibility to obesity and metabolic disorders in adulthood, highlighting the lasting impact of early environmental influences on genetic expression.

Natural selection has played a pivotal role in shaping genetic traits related to body composition. Throughout human evolution, populations have faced varying environmental pressures that influenced the selection of genes associated with energy storage and metabolism. For instance, in environments where food scarcity was common, genes promoting efficient fat storage would have conferred a survival advantage. Conversely, in environments with abundant food resources, the selective pressure for such genes would be reduced. This evolutionary perspective helps explain the prevalence of certain obesity-related genes in modern populations.

The rapid evolution of the U.S. population over the past 250 years provides a compelling case study for understanding the interaction between genetics and environmental changes. The initial immigrant population, fleeing famine and scarcity, faced different selective pressures compared to contemporary society, characterised by food abundance and sedentary lifestyles. This shift has likely contributed to the high prevalence of obesity in the U.S. today. Studies suggest that the genetic predisposition to store fat, which was advantageous in times of scarcity, has become maladaptive in the context of modern dietary and lifestyle patterns.

Specific genes have been linked to obesity and body fat distribution, providing insights into the underlying biological mechanisms. The melanocortin 4 receptor (MC4R) gene is one such example. Mutations in MC4R are the most common monogenic cause of severe obesity, affecting the regulation of appetite and energy balance. Individuals with MC4R mutations exhibit hyperphagia (excessive eating) and reduced energy expenditure, leading to significant weight gain. Another gene, the peroxisome proliferator-activated receptor gamma (PPARG), plays a crucial role in adipocyte differentiation and lipid metabolism. Variants in PPARG are associated with differences in fat distribution and the risk of metabolic syndrome. The study of epigenetics has further illuminated the complex relationship between genes and body composition. Research on the agouti viable yellow (Avy) mouse model has demonstrated how maternal diet can influence the epigenetic regulation of genes involved in obesity. When pregnant Avy mice were fed a diet rich in methyl donors, the offspring exhibited lower levels of obesity and metabolic disorders. This finding underscores the potential for dietary interventions to modify epigenetic marks and alter the risk of obesity.

Epigenetic research on human populations has revealed similar patterns. For instance, a study by Heijmans et al. (2008) investigated the epigenetic effects of prenatal exposure to the Dutch Famine. The researchers found persistent changes in DNA methylation at specific loci associated with metabolic health in individuals exposed to famine in utero. These epigenetic alterations were linked to increased susceptibility to obesity and other metabolic disorders, providing a mechanistic explanation for the long-term health effects of prenatal malnutrition.

The interplay between genetics and environment is further exemplified by the concept of gene-environment interactions. Certain genetic variants may increase an individual's susceptibility to obesity only in the presence of specific environmental factors. For example, individuals with variants in the FTO gene are more likely to gain weight when exposed to high-fat, high-calorie diets. This interaction highlights the importance of considering both genetic and environmental factors in addressing obesity and related health issues.

James Watson and Francis Crick discovered the double-helix structure of DNA in 1953, which provided some insight into how mutations could develop spontaneously. The scientists' landmark article demonstrated that when DNA was copied, specific letters of the genetic code could be substituted for others. Adenine can be replaced with guanine (or vice versa), and cytosine with thymine. However, numerous other types of faults could arise. The insertion or deletion of chemical letters may cause the DNA sequence to lengthen or shorten. Accidentally copying entire areas may occur. Sequences may be cut and pasted elsewhere. Errors in the production of egg or sperm cells can result in an embryo with an extra chromosome, as seen in Down syndrome, where a kid inherits a third copy of chromosome 21. The most drastic modifications entail inheriting an additional copy of the whole genome, which might start as a malfunction in egg or sperm production.

The role of genetics in body composition is also relevant to evolutionary biology. Studies on insular vertebrates, for example, have shown how isolation on islands can lead to rapid evolutionary changes in body size. The phenomenon, known as the "island rule," suggests that small-bodied species tend to evolve larger sizes on islands, while large-bodied species evolve smaller sizes. This pattern reflects the selective pressures of limited resources and reduced predation, providing insights into how environmental factors drive genetic adaptations.

Human populations have also experienced similar evolutionary pressures. The transition from hunter-gatherer societies to agricultural and industrialised societies brought significant changes in diet and lifestyle. These shifts likely influenced the selection of genes related to energy metabolism and fat storage. For example, the "thrifty gene" hypothesis posits that genes promoting efficient energy storage were advantageous during periods of food scarcity but have become detrimental in modern environments with constant food availability.

Case studies of specific genes provide a deeper understanding of the genetic basis for body composition. The MC4R gene, as mentioned earlier, is a prime example. Individuals with MC4R mutations often exhibit severe early-onset obesity, highlighting the critical role of this gene in regulating energy balance. Another gene, the adiponectin gene (ADIPOQ), is associated with adiponectin levels, a hormone involved in glucose regulation and fatty acid oxidation. Variants in ADIPOQ influence body fat distribution and the risk of metabolic disorders, demonstrating the complex genetic regulation of adiposity. The study of body composition genetics is not limited to obesity. Genetic factors also influence other aspects of body size and shape, such as height and muscle mass. For instance, the growth hormone receptor (GHR) gene plays a crucial role in determining height by regulating the effects of growth hormone. Variants in GHR are associated with differences in stature, providing insights into the genetic basis of height variation.

Similarly, the myostatin (MSTN) gene, which inhibits muscle growth, has been studied extensively in relation to muscle mass and strength. Mutations in MSTN result in increased muscle mass and strength, as observed in both humans and animals. This gene has potential therapeutic implications for conditions characterised by muscle wasting, such as muscular dystrophy.

The genetic basis for body composition is a complex and multifaceted field that encompasses the interplay between numerous genes, environmental factors, and evolutionary pressures. Scientific studies and statistical data provide robust evidence for the significant genetic contribution to body size, shape, and body fat mass index. The inheritance of these traits is influenced by a combination of genetic variants, epigenetic modifications, and gene-environment interactions. Understanding these mechanisms is crucial for developing targeted interventions and treatments for obesity and related health issues, as well as for advancing our knowledge of human evolution and adaptation. The rapid evolution of the U.S. population, driven by changes in diet and lifestyle, exemplifies the dynamic nature of genetic and environmental interactions in shaping body composition.

Human genetics, like the rest of modern biology, is a materialist science that sees the body and living processes as the product of chemical and physical laws. However, research has demonstrated that genes do not function in the same way that computer programs do, when they are left to crunch numbers while a programmer sleeps. Cells and organisms always respond to their surroundings. The weather and natural terrain, the smog above a metropolis, a person's cubicle, cramped aeroplane seats, and the toxins in drinking water are all part of the human environment, as are human civilisation, science, the Internet, music, and ideas.

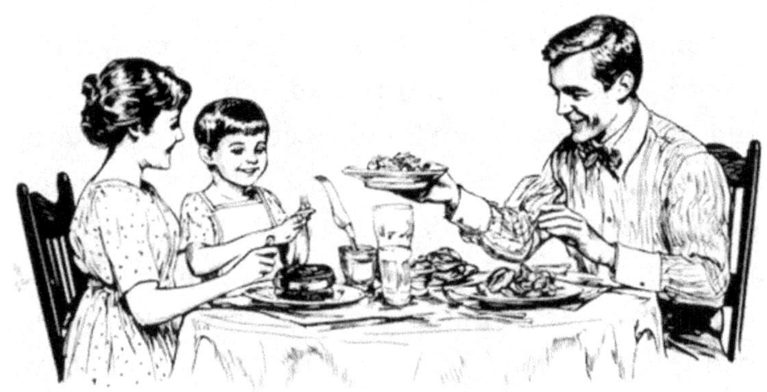

4. The US Population

The complex nature of human body composition is significantly influenced by various environmental factors. These include diet, lifestyle, and socio-economic status, all of which play a crucial role in shaping individuals' physicality. A major part of this influence stems from the environment in which individuals live and the resources available to them. The modern American food environment, characterized by the abundance, variety, and affordability of high-carbohydrate and sugary foods, has profoundly impacted body composition. Over the past 250 years, dietary patterns and lifestyles have dramatically shifted, resulting in significant changes in body composition.

The American food environment has evolved drastically from the colonial period to the present day. In the 18th and early 19th centuries, the average American diet was based on subsistence farming, with families growing their own food and relying heavily on vegetables, grains, and occasional meat. This diet was high in fibre and low in refined sugars and fats. The Industrial Revolution in the mid-19th century led to a gradual shift as food production became industrialised, introducing processed foods and mass production. However, it was not until the mid-20th century that the American food landscape underwent a significant transformation. The post-World War II era saw the rise of convenience foods, fast food restaurants, and a dramatic increase in the consumption of high-calorie, low-nutrient foods. The introduction of high-fructose corn syrup in the 1970s further exacerbated the shift towards a diet high in sugars and refined carbohydrates.

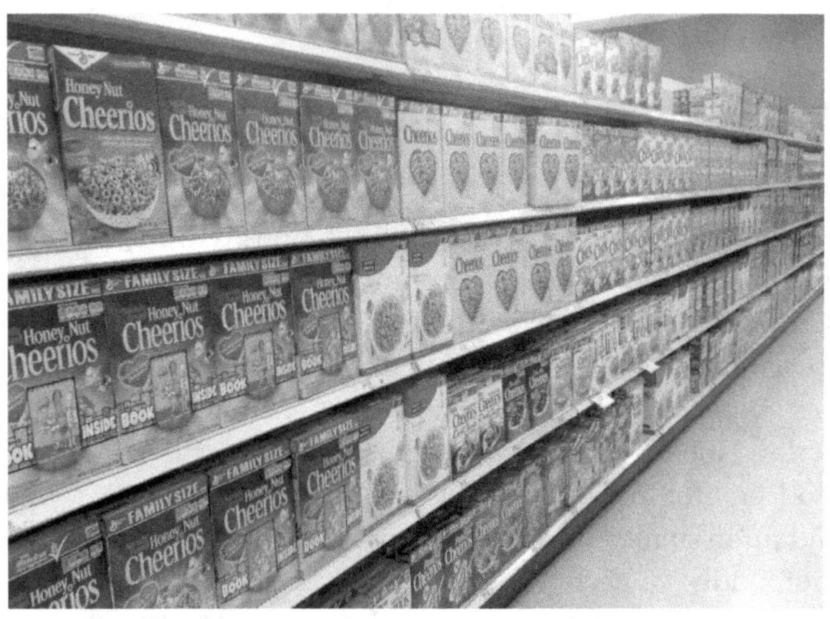

This transformation in the food environment has been accompanied by significant lifestyle changes. Technological advancements and the rise of sedentary occupations have decreased physical activity. In the past, daily life involved significant physical exertion through farming, manual labour, or domestic chores. Today, the prevalence of desk jobs, automobiles, and screen-based entertainment has drastically reduced physical activity. This sedentary lifestyle, combined with the increased availability of high-calorie foods, has led to a rise in caloric consumption without a corresponding increase in energy expenditure.

Socio-economic status also plays a crucial role in shaping body composition. Access to healthy food options is often limited in lower-income neighbourhoods, where convenience stores and fast-food restaurants are more prevalent than grocery stores offering fresh produce. These areas, known as food deserts, create environments where high-calorie, nutrient-poor foods are the most accessible option. Economic constraints often force individuals to opt for cheaper, calorie-dense foods rather than more expensive, nutritious options. This socio-economic disparity in diet quality significantly contributes to differences in body composition across various socio-economic groups.

One of the most striking examples of environmental factors' impact on body composition is the rapid increase in obesity rates in the United States. According to the Centers for Disease Control and Prevention (CDC), the prevalence of obesity among adults in the United States was approximately 15% in the 1970s. By 2020, this figure had risen to over 40%. This increase cannot be attributed solely to genetic factors, as the genetic makeup of the population has not changed significantly in such a short period. Instead, it highlights the powerful influence of environmental factors such as diet and lifestyle.

The impact of diet on body composition is well-documented. Diets high in refined sugars and carbohydrates lead to increased fat storage and weight gain. High-carbohydrate diets cause rapid spikes in blood sugar levels, prompting the release of insulin, which facilitates fat storage. Over time, this can lead to insulin resistance and metabolic disorders such as type 2 diabetes. In contrast, diets rich in whole foods, including vegetables, fruits, lean proteins, and whole grains, are associated with healthier body composition and a lower risk of chronic diseases. The Mediterranean diet, for example, which emphasises whole foods and healthy fats, has been shown to promote weight loss and improve metabolic health.

Lifestyle factors such as physical activity also play a critical role in determining body composition. Regular physical activity increases energy expenditure, helping to maintain a healthy weight and reduce body fat. Exercise also has numerous other health benefits, including improved cardiovascular health, enhanced mood, and better metabolic function. Sedentary behaviour, on the other hand, is associated with weight gain and an increased risk of obesity and related health problems. The rise of sedentary lifestyles in the United States is a significant contributor to the obesity epidemic.

The interaction between genetic factors and environmental influences is complex and multifaceted. While genetic predisposition plays a significant role in determining body size and shape, environmental factors such as diet and lifestyle can modulate genetic expression. This interaction is the focus of the field of epigenetics, which studies how environmental factors can influence gene expression without changing the underlying DNA sequence. Epigenetic changes can be induced by factors such as diet, physical activity, and exposure to toxins, and can have lasting effects on health and body composition.

When considering how genetic engineering could be utilised to enhance our lot as humans, we must fully understand the complexity and repercussions. One day in the near future, we shall be able to intervene in our own growth. This would entail making a decision: whether to prioritise some genetic features over others. The challenges surrounding this topic are both moral and technical: much more needs to be learnt about the interactions between genes and the environment before we can effectively alter our hereditary material, assuming individuals feel it is desirable to do so.

The rapid changes in the food environment and lifestyle in the United States over the past 250 years provide a compelling case study of how environmental factors can influence body composition. The shift from a subsistence-based diet to one dominated by processed foods and high in sugars and refined carbohydrates, combined with a decrease in physical activity, has led to a dramatic increase in obesity rates and related health problems. Understanding the interplay between genetic and environmental factors is crucial for developing effective strategies to combat obesity and promote healthy body composition.

The environmental influence on body composition is profound and multifaceted. The American food environment, characterised by an abundance of high-carbohydrate and sugary foods, has played a significant role in shaping body composition. Lifestyle changes, including increased sedentary behaviour and higher caloric intake, have further exacerbated the issue. Socio-economic status also plays a critical role, with lower-income individuals often facing limited access to healthy food options. The rapid increase in obesity rates in the United States highlights the powerful impact of environmental factors on body composition. While genetic predisposition is a significant factor, the interaction between genes and environment, as studied in the field of epigenetics, provides valuable insights into how environmental influences can modulate genetic expression and impact health. The history of the American food environment and lifestyle changes over the past 250 years offers a compelling example of how environmental factors can shape body composition, underscoring the importance of addressing these factors to promote health and well-being.

The theory of rapid evolution and adaptation in response to an environment of food abundance explores the intersection of genetics, environmental pressures, and human physiology. Rapid evolution refers to the relatively swift genetic changes that can occur within populations over a few generations, influenced by selective pressures such as food availability. This concept is particularly pertinent in the context of the United States over the past 250 years, where an immigrant population fleeing famine conditions in Europe encountered an environment of unprecedented food abundance.

As immigrants settled in the United States during the 18th and 19th centuries, they encountered an environment vastly different from their homelands. Europe had been marked by periods of famine and food scarcity, shaping the physiological and genetic traits of its populations. Many immigrants came from regions where the struggle for survival had selected for traits that favoured energy conservation and efficient food utilisation, often referred to as "thrifty genes." These genes are theorised to enhance fat storage and minimise energy expenditure, traits advantageous in environments where food was unpredictable.

In the new environment of America, however, the constant availability of food presented a stark contrast. This abundance removed the selective pressure for energy conservation, leading to significant changes in the population's body composition over successive generations. Studies suggest that the human body can undergo notable physiological changes in response to consistent food availability, altering not only metabolic rates but also the predisposition to store fat.

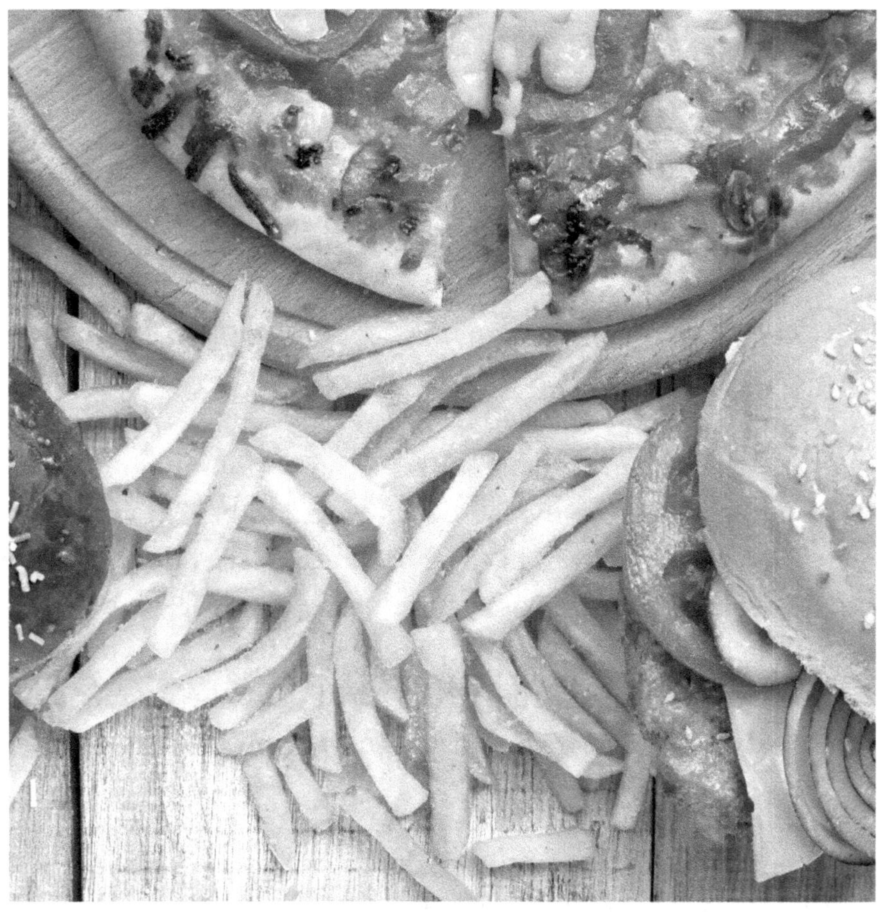

The concept of "thrifty genes" was first introduced by geneticist James Neel in 1962. Neel hypothesised that certain populations evolved genetic mechanisms to efficiently store fat during periods of food scarcity, which would then be advantageous during times of famine. However, in environments of food abundance, these same genetic traits could predispose individuals to obesity and related metabolic disorders. The United States, with its rapid transition to an environment of food abundance, provides a living laboratory for examining these evolutionary dynamics.

Over approximately six generations, the American population has exhibited remarkable adaptations to its environment. Data show a significant increase in average body mass index (BMI) and body fat percentage. This trend can be attributed to the gradual adaptation between genetic predispositions and environmental factors. The availability of calorie-dense foods, coupled with a sedentary lifestyle, has accentuated the expression of thrifty genes, leading to higher rates of obesity.

Every human person contains inside his or her cells a long history of the species. The human genome is a record of evolution that dates back to the first Homo sapiens and beyond, to the earliest primates, animals, and the beginnings of life itself. Human genetics is the study of such information and its application to people's lives — how their bodies develop, how they behave, whether they are healthy or sick, and other elements of human existence that genes influence. It is the study of how genes transfer from one generation to the next. It is also the study of human DNA's origins and changes across time.

Another aspect of the research by Tessa J. Roseboom and colleagues on the Dutch Hunger Winter has shown that individuals exposed to famine in utero tend to have higher rates of obesity, diabetes, and cardiovascular disease in later life. These findings suggest that the prenatal environment can programme metabolic traits, making individuals more susceptible to obesity when exposed to food abundance later in life. Similar patterns have been observed in populations that experienced famine conditions in Russia, reinforcing the idea that genetic and epigenetic mechanisms are at play.

The comparison between the United States and Russia illustrates how different environments can shape genetic and physiological traits. In the U.S., the shift to food abundance has led to an increased prevalence of obesity and metabolic disorders, as the once advantageous thrifty genes become maladaptive. Conversely, in Russia, ongoing periods of food scarcity continue to favour the retention of these genes, resulting in different body composition and health outcomes.

The concept of "thrifty genes" is further supported by epigenetic research, which examines how environmental factors can alter gene expression without changing the underlying DNA sequence. Epigenetics plays a crucial role in how genes are expressed in response to environmental conditions, such as diet and lifestyle. For instance, research by Heijmans and colleagues on the epigenetic effects of the Dutch Hunger Winter has demonstrated that prenatal exposure to famine can lead to persistent changes in DNA methylation, a key epigenetic mechanism. These changes can affect metabolic pathways and increase the risk of obesity and related diseases in later life.

The role of epigenetics in rapid evolution is profound, as it allows for quick adaptations to environmental changes across generations. Unlike genetic mutations, which occur slowly over many generations, epigenetic changes can happen within a single generation and be passed down to offspring. This mechanism provides a way for populations to rapidly adapt to new environments, such as the transition from food scarcity to abundance.

In the context of the United States, the transition from a population of immigrants fleeing famine to one of the most obese populations in the world can be seen as a case study in rapid evolution. The constant availability of food has shifted the selective pressures, favouring traits that predispose individuals to higher body fat. This shift is evident in the rising rates of obesity, diabetes, and other metabolic disorders.

Of course, there is still much to learn in each subject, and the various perspectives on human nature that they offer are far from united. The image will not be complete until researchers get a much greater knowledge of the brain, which includes phenomena such as memory and learning, awareness, dreams, and spiritual experiences. Nonetheless, there is something amazing about this science going forward in the twenty-first century: genetics, evolution, cell biology, embryology, chemistry, and medicine are beginning to present a coherent picture of the biological aspect of human existence.

The theory of rapid evolution and adaptation in response to an environment of food abundance provides a compelling framework for understanding the changes in the U.S. population over the past 250 years. The interplay between thrifty genes, epigenetic mechanisms, and environmental factors has driven significant changes in body composition and health outcomes. By comparing these trends with populations in food-deprived regions, such as Russia, we can gain a deeper understanding of how different evolutionary pressures shape genetic and physiological traits. This knowledge is essential for developing effective strategies to address the public health implications of obesity and related metabolic disorders in modern societies.

Exploring the empirical evidence regarding body composition trends within the U.S. population over the past 250 years reveals a fascinating unique and well documented field of study, between genetics, dietary habits, and environmental factors. The theory positing that approximately 70% of human body size, shape, and body fat mass index is genetically predetermined, while the remaining 30% is influenced by lifestyle and diet, finds substantial support in both historical and contemporary data. This theory underscores the rapid evolutionary changes witnessed in the U.S. population, evolving from an initial immigrant population facing famine to one characterised by high obesity rates. This shift can largely be attributed to the genetic response to food abundance over generations.

The historical context of the U.S. population provides a rich tapestry for examining changes in body composition. The initial settlers, primarily European immigrants fleeing famine and seeking better opportunities, brought with them genetic predispositions shaped by centuries of scarcity. These predispositions included thrifty genes, which are advantageous in environments where food is scarce but become detrimental in contexts of abundance. Over time, as the U.S. transformed into a land of plenty, these genetic traits contributed to rising obesity rates.

Statistical analysis of obesity rates and body composition trends in the U.S. reveals a marked increase in obesity over the past few decades. According to data from the Centres for Disease Control and Prevention (CDC), the prevalence of obesity among U.S. adults has more than doubled since the 1960s. In 1960, approximately 13% of adults were classified as obese, whereas recent estimates indicate that over 42% of adults fall into this category. This dramatic rise is mirrored in children and adolescents, with current statistics showing that nearly 20% of youths are obese, compared to less than 5% in the 1960s. This increase in obesity rates can be attributed to a combination of genetic factors, dietary changes, and a more sedentary lifestyle.

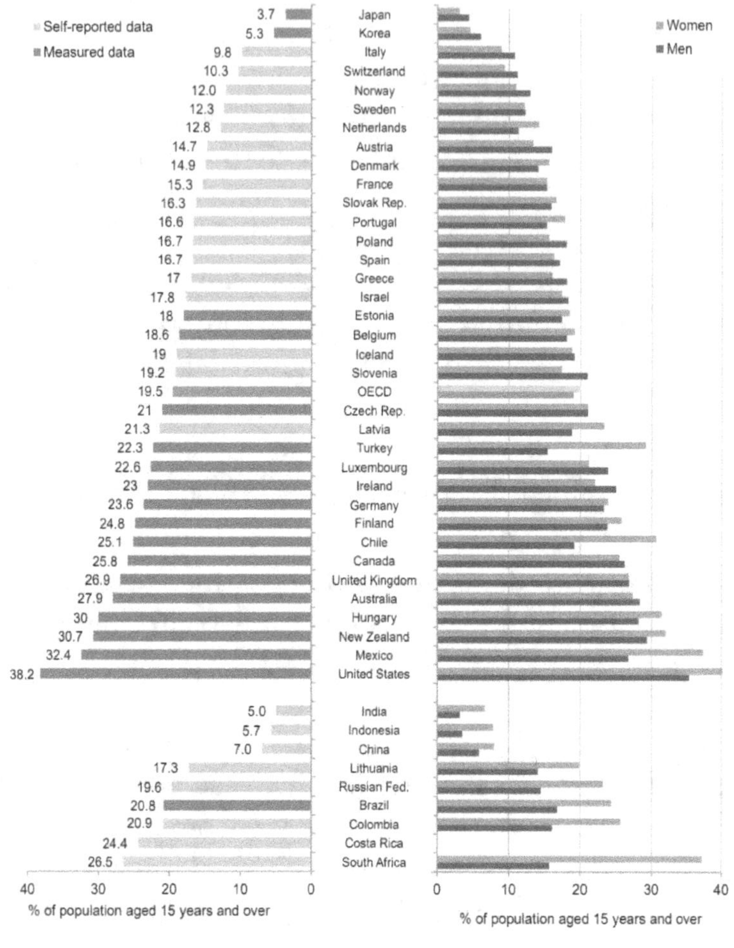

The examination of body composition trends across different demographic groups within the U.S. provides further insights into the complex relationship of genetics and environment. For instance, obesity rates vary significantly among racial and ethnic groups. Non-Hispanic Black adults have the highest prevalence of obesity (49.6%), followed by Hispanic adults (44.8%), non-Hispanic White adults (42.2%), and non-Hispanic Asian adults (17.4%). These disparities are influenced by a variety of factors, including socio-economic status, cultural dietary practices, and access to healthcare and recreational facilities. Additionally, genetic differences among these groups can predispose certain populations to higher obesity rates, as discussed in studies like those by O'Rahilly and Farooqi (2008), which highlight the heritable aspects of obesity and its sensitivity to environmental conditions.

Longitudinal studies tracking changes in body composition across generations provide compelling evidence of the genetic and environmental influences on obesity. For example, the Framingham Heart Study, which began in 1948, has followed multiple generations of participants to investigate the factors contributing to cardiovascular disease. This study has revealed that offspring of obese parents are significantly more likely to be obese themselves, underscoring the hereditary nature of obesity. Moreover, these longitudinal studies have shown that environmental changes, such as increased availability of high-calorie foods and decreased physical activity, have exacerbated genetic predispositions to obesity in subsequent generations.

The role of epigenetics in shaping body composition is also crucial to understanding the rapid evolution of the U.S. population. Epigenetic changes, which involve modifications to gene expression without altering the DNA sequence, can be triggered by environmental factors such as diet and stress. These changes can be passed down through generations, contributing to the observed trends in obesity. Studies like those by Weaver et al. (2004) have demonstrated how maternal behaviour can epigenetically programme offspring, influencing their metabolic health and susceptibility to obesity. This epigenetic inheritance helps explain how the U.S. population, initially predisposed to withstand famine, has adapted to an environment of food abundance with increasing rates of obesity.

The transition from a population facing food scarcity to one characterised by food overabundance has profound implications for public health. The abundance of high-calorie, nutrient-poor foods, combined with a sedentary lifestyle, has created an environment conducive to obesity. This shift is evident in the dietary patterns of the U.S. population, where processed foods and sugary beverages have become staples. The influence of these dietary habits on body composition is significant, as demonstrated by the work of researchers like Taubes (2010), who highlights the impact of carbohydrate consumption on insulin resistance and fat accumulation.

The empirical evidence from the U.S. population over the past 250 years supports the theory that genetic factors play a predominant role in determining body size, shape, and fat mass index, while dietary and lifestyle factors contribute significantly to these traits. The rapid evolution of the U.S. population from famine-stricken immigrants to one of the most obese populations globally illustrates the dynamic adaptations that all species and not least humans can undergo in response to dramatic changes in environmental conditions. Longitudinal studies, statistical analyses, and research on epigenetics provide a comprehensive understanding of how these factors have shaped body composition trends in the U.S., highlighting the importance of considering both genetic predispositions and environmental influences in addressing the obesity epidemic. This exploration underscores the complexity of human evolution and adaptation, offering valuable insights for public health initiatives aimed at mitigating the impacts of obesity on future generations.

The human body's evolutionary trajectory has been marked by a significant increase in body fat mass, a trend driven by a combination of genetic, environmental, and behavioural factors. Reversing this evolutionary trend presents an intricate challenge that requires a multifaceted approach. The feasibility of achieving such a reversal hinges on our understanding of genetic predispositions, the implementation of effective public health policies, and the promotion of dietary and lifestyle interventions.

Genetic predisposition plays a critical role in determining body composition. Studies indicate that approximately 70% of human body size, shape, and fat mass index is predetermined by genetic factors. This assertion is supported by research in gene memory, epigenetics, and rapid evolutionary changes observed in both humans and animals. For instance, the U.S. population has undergone significant changes over the past 250 years, evolving from an immigrant population fleeing famine to one of the most obese populations in the world. This rapid evolution can largely be attributed to the abundance of food and the genetic response to this abundance over numerous generations.

Human genetics, like the rest of modern biology, is a materialist science that sees the body and living processes as the product of chemical and physical laws. However, research has demonstrated that genes do not function in the same way that computer programs do, when they are left to crunch numbers while a programmer sleeps. Cells and organisms always respond to their surroundings. The weather and natural terrain, the smog above a metropolis, a person's cubicle, cramped aeroplane seats, and the toxins in drinking water are all part of the human environment, as are human civilisation, science, the Internet, music, and ideas. British biologist Stephen Rose stated it this way: "I don't think we can grasp what it means to be human until we recognise that we are evolved beings as well as social, historical, cultural, and technological entities.

Public health policies aimed at reducing obesity rates must address both genetic predispositions and environmental factors. Policies that promote access to healthy foods, regulate the marketing of high-calorie, low-nutrient foods, and encourage physical activity are essential. For example, Finland's North Karelia Project, initiated in the 1970s, successfully reduced cardiovascular disease and obesity rates through comprehensive community-based interventions. These included dietary changes, smoking cessation programmes, and increased physical activity, demonstrating that sustained public health efforts can lead to significant improvements in population health.

Lifestyle changes, including increased physical activity and behavioural modifications, are also vital. Regular exercise has been shown to improve metabolic health and reduce body fat, even in individuals with a genetic predisposition to obesity. Programmes that encourage active transportation, such as biking and walking, and provide access to recreational facilities can help promote a more active lifestyle. Additionally, behavioural interventions that address emotional and psychological factors related to eating can be effective in achieving long-term weight management.

The time frame required for significant changes in body composition varies depending on genetic predisposition and the extent of environmental and behavioural modifications. While some individuals may experience rapid improvements, others may require sustained efforts over several years or even generations to achieve significant changes. Epigenetic research, as discussed by Weaver et al. (2004), suggests that modifications in gene expression can occur relatively quickly in response to environmental changes, but reversing deeply ingrained genetic predispositions may take longer.

Case studies of populations that have successfully reduced obesity rates through sustained efforts provide valuable insights into the feasibility of reversing the trend of increased body fat mass. Japan, for example, has one of the lowest obesity rates in the world, attributed to a combination of traditional dietary patterns, high levels of physical activity, and robust public health policies. The traditional Japanese diet, which emphasises fish, vegetables, and rice, combined with cultural practices that encourage physical activity, has contributed to the population's overall health and low obesity rates.

As discussed earlier Pacific Island nations have experienced a dramatic rise in obesity rates due to the rapid adoption of Western dietary patterns and sedentary lifestyles. Efforts to reverse this trend have focused on promoting traditional diets and increasing physical activity. For instance, Samoa has implemented community-based programmes to reintroduce traditional foods and encourage physical activity, resulting in gradual improvements in obesity rates and overall health.

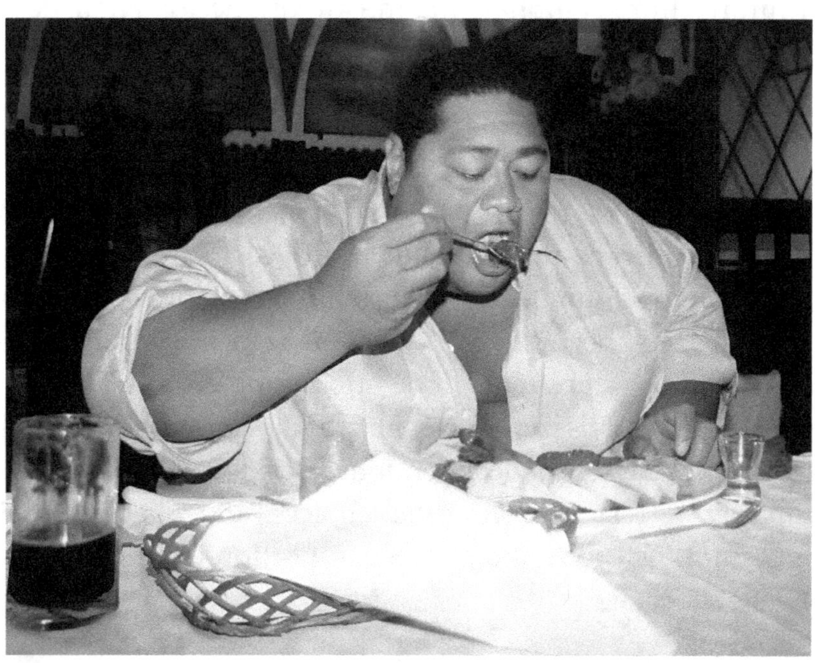

The feasibility of reversing the evolutionary trend of increased body fat mass is complex and multifaceted, requiring a combination of genetic, environmental, and behavioural interventions. While genetic predisposition plays a significant role, public health policies, dietary interventions, and lifestyle changes are crucial in achieving these goals. The time frame for significant changes varies, but sustained efforts over multiple generations may be necessary to achieve lasting improvements. Case studies from various populations highlight the potential for success through comprehensive and sustained efforts, offering valuable lessons for global public health strategies.

In summary, the challenge of reversing the evolutionary trend of increased body fat mass is formidable but not insurmountable. By understanding the genetic underpinnings of obesity and implementing effective public health policies, dietary interventions, and lifestyle changes, it is possible to make significant strides in improving population health. The lessons learned from successful case studies provide a roadmap for future efforts, emphasising the importance of a holistic and sustained approach to addressing the obesity epidemic.

The implications of the genetic predisposition theory for public health and obesity prevention are vast and multifaceted. As the understanding of how genetics influence body composition deepens, the public health sector is compelled to re-evaluate traditional approaches to obesity prevention. This shift in perspective is essential given that genetic predispositions account for approximately 70% of an individual's body size, shape, and body fat mass index. This theory challenges the conventional wisdom that obesity is primarily a result of lifestyle choices and dietary habits, suggesting instead that a significant portion is predetermined by genetic factors.

One major implication for public health is the need for more personalised and targeted interventions. Traditional obesity prevention programmes often employ a one-size-fits-all approach, focusing on generalised dietary guidelines and exercise routines. However, the recognition of genetic predispositions necessitates a more nuanced strategy. Personalised medicine, which tailors' health interventions to individual genetic profiles, emerges as a promising avenue. This approach could lead to more effective prevention and treatment plans by considering an individual's genetic makeup alongside their lifestyle and environmental factors.

Genetic counselling also becomes increasingly important in this context. By providing individuals with information about their genetic predispositions, genetic counselling can help them make informed decisions about their health. For instance, those with a genetic predisposition to obesity could benefit from early interventions and continuous monitoring, reducing their risk of developing related health issues such as diabetes, cardiovascular diseases, and certain cancers. Genetic counselling thus becomes a critical tool in empowering individuals to take proactive measures in managing their health.

The exploration of potential future research directions and perhaps led by you dear genius reader will be significant. To further understand the genetic and environmental factors influencing body composition, multidisciplinary research efforts are required. Studies integrating genetics, epigenetics, nutrition, and behavioural sciences could uncover the complex interplay between genes and environment. For instance, research into epigenetics—how gene expression is influenced by environmental factors such as diet, stress, and physical activity—holds great promise. The works of Heijmans et al.

(2008) and Weaver et al. (2004) highlight the persistent epigenetic differences associated with prenatal exposure to famine and maternal behaviour, respectively. These findings suggest that early-life environmental factors can have long-lasting effects on an individual's genetic expression and, consequently, their propensity for obesity.

A child inherits a body with unique features from their parents, but without a user manual. Creating such a documentation for a machine requires a comprehensive technical description of the system's components, functions, and interdependence. Our DNA and Biology does something similar and provides a detailed account of the body plan a bit like a design manual. However, our DNA cannot write the guidebook; it is the responsibility of scientists and researchers to understand why variations may occurs, and hopefully this book will provide some smart genius with spark of ingenuity to delve into this research.

Future research should also focus on the evolutionary aspects of body size and obesity. The rapid evolution of the U.S. population over the past 250 years, transitioning from an immigrant population fleeing famine to one of the most obese populations globally, exemplifies the impact of environmental abundance on genetic adaptation. Studies on body size evolution in insular vertebrates, as discussed by Lomolino (2005) and Van der Knaap (1996), can provide analogies for understanding human obesity. These studies suggest that isolation and resource availability play crucial roles in shaping body size, which can be extrapolated to human populations experiencing rapid changes in diet and lifestyle.

Ethical considerations and societal impacts are paramount when focusing on genetic predisposition in obesity research and interventions. One ethical concern is the potential for genetic determinism—the belief that genes alone dictate health outcomes. Such a perspective could lead to fatalism, where individuals feel powerless to change their health status. It is crucial to communicate that while genetics play a significant role, lifestyle and environmental factors still have a substantial impact. Public health messages should emphasise that genetic predisposition is not destiny and that healthy behaviours can mitigate genetic risks.

Moreover, there is a risk of stigmatisation and discrimination based on genetic information. Individuals identified as having a genetic predisposition to obesity might face prejudice in employment, insurance, and social interactions. Therefore, robust privacy protections and anti-discrimination laws are essential to safeguard individuals' genetic information. Ethical guidelines must ensure that genetic data is used responsibly and that individuals are not unfairly penalised for their genetic makeup.

The societal impacts of focusing on genetic predisposition are also profound. On one hand, acknowledging the genetic basis of obesity can reduce stigma by shifting the narrative away from personal blame and towards a more compassionate understanding of the condition. On the other hand, it necessitates a reallocation of public health resources to support genetic research and personalised interventions. This shift could lead to disparities in access to advanced genetic testing and personalised healthcare, particularly in underserved communities. Ensuring equitable access to these innovations is a critical challenge that policymakers must address.

The genetic predisposition theory has far-reaching implications for public health and obesity prevention. It calls for a paradigm shift towards personalised medicine and genetic counselling, recognising the complex interplay between genetics and environment. Future research must continue to unravel the genetic and epigenetic mechanisms underlying body composition, informed by historical and evolutionary perspectives. Ethical considerations and societal impacts must be carefully navigated to ensure that genetic information is used to empower individuals and promote health equity. As the scientific community delves deeper into the genetic underpinnings of obesity, it is imperative to maintain a balanced and inclusive approach, ensuring that the benefits of this knowledge are accessible to all.

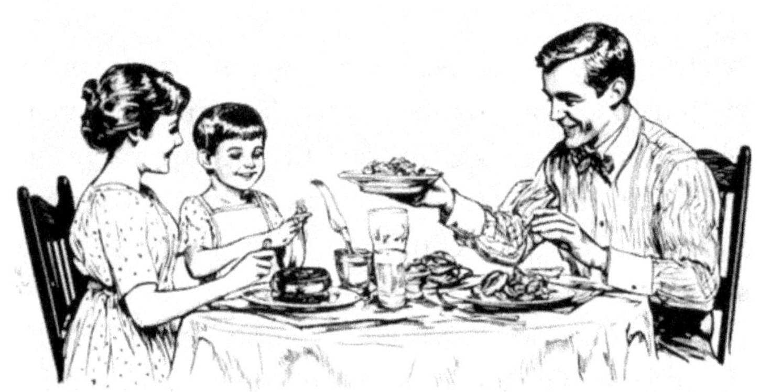

5. Genes in brief

The human ACTN3 gene produces a protein called alpha-actinin-3, essential for muscle structure and metabolism. This gene can undergo a variation known as a single nucleotide polymorphism (SNP) at a specific location, changing an arginine (R) to a stop codon (X). The R allele represents the normal, functional version of the gene, while the X allele stops the production of functional alpha-actinin-3 protein.

This genetic variation, known as the ACTN3 R577X polymorphism, is associated with differences in athletic performance, particularly in power sports like track and field events. A study examined the prevalence of these gene variations among runners, swimmers, and non-athletes to understand this association better.

The study included 137 runners, 91 swimmers, and 217 non-athletes. Runners were divided into long-distance (LDR) and short-distance (SDR) groups, while swimmers were categorised into long-distance (LDS) and short-distance (SDS) groups. Genomic DNA was extracted from blood samples, and genotypes were determined using a specific assay.

The results revealed significant differences in genotypes among runners. Long-distance runners had the lowest prevalence of the RR genotype and the R allele, but a higher prevalence of the XX genotype and X allele. Conversely, there were no significant differences in genotype and allele frequencies between LDS and SDS swimmers. However, LDS had higher frequencies of the RR genotype and R allele compared to LDR.

This suggests that the ACTN3 R577X polymorphism can distinguish between short-distance and long-distance runners but is less effective in differentiating between short-distance and long-distance swimmers.

Alpha-actinin-3 is crucial in fast-twitch muscle fibres, which are vital for high-intensity muscle contractions. This protein is encoded by the ACTN3 gene, which can have a polymorphism affecting its production. Individuals with the RR genotype (two R alleles) and RX heterozygotes (one R and one X allele) produce functional alpha-actinin-3, while those with the XX genotype (two X alleles) do not.

Research indicates that the ACTN3 genotype is linked to athletic performance, with higher frequencies of the R allele found in elite and professional sprint and power athletes compared to the general population. For example, hypothetically, if 95% of male 100m Olympic medallists had the RR genotype, it would suggest a genetic advantage in power-based sports.

In a specific study involving professional badminton players, the ACTN3 RR genotype was most common, with 49.1% having this genotype, 22.6% being RX, and 28.3% having the XX genotype. Notably, none of the top ten ranked badminton players had the XX genotype. This suggests that having the RR or RX genotype might confer an advantage in reaching elite levels in badminton, characterised by high-intensity actions like rapid direction changes, accelerations, jumps, and smashes.

Compared to the general European population, the distribution of the ACTN3 genotypes in badminton players showed a higher prevalence of the RR genotype and a lower prevalence of the RX genotype, indicating a possible genetic advantage.

ACTN3 Genotypes

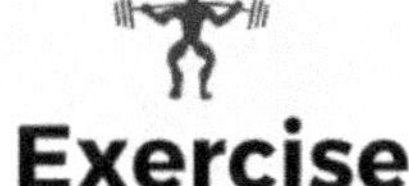

Exercise

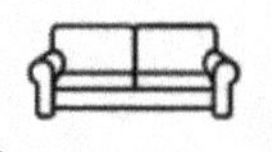

Recovery

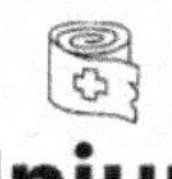

Injury

R allele
(C/C or C/T genotype)
Better response to resistance training

R allele
(C/C or C/T genotype)
Less muscle damage from eccentric training

R allele
(C/C or C/T genotype)
Lower risk of injuries

XX genotype
(TT genotype)
Less response to resistance training

XX genotype
(TT genotype)
More muscle damage from eccentric training

XX genotype
(TT genotype)
Higher injury risk

The presence of functional alpha-actinin-3, associated with the RR and RX genotypes of the ACTN3 gene, appears to provide an advantage in becoming an elite athlete in power-based disciplines such as sprinting and possibly in sports like badminton. Large-scale studies across different ethnic backgrounds are needed to confirm the association of the R allele of ACTN3 with performance in various sports. However, from the limited studies so far, there is a lot of evidence suggesting that athletes with a West African ancestral origin for example countries like Nigeria, Sierra Leon etc, still carry the RR genotype. Hence the success of athletes in countries like the US, Jamaica & Caribbean countries in sprinting and other events where explosive power is required.

Whereas athletes with an East African ancestral origin, for example Ethiopia & Kenya, living and having to adapt to a hunter gatherer lifestyle on the wide open plains where the emphasis is on stamina and endurance, the RR genotype is no longer present in those populations.

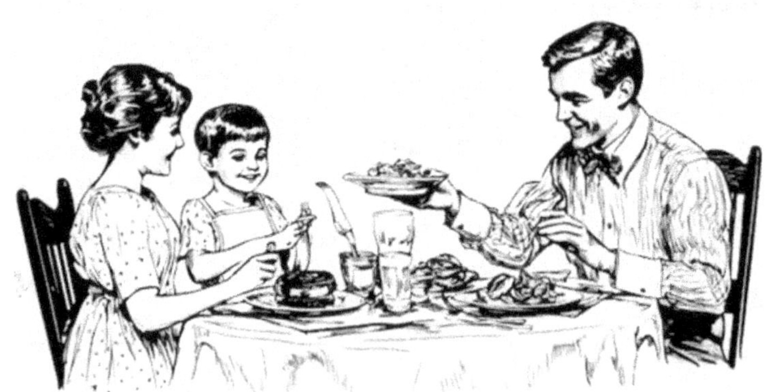

6. Losing weight in your lifetime.

Hopefully the explanations given in the preceding chapters have provided sufficient evidence to suggest, that in order for an obese person to lose weight permanently in their lifetime whilst possible, you will always be battling against how you have been built, genetically. You will always feel hungry and want to fill that large stomach that your body plan has provided for you. It does work both ways, the skinny person that might fat shame you have never had to work really hard to keep their weight down, and no amount of whey protein is going to turn them into the Rock. In fact, there are some famous puny fat shamers who would find it physically impossible to say put on four stones in weight, they are simply descended from the wrong people.

You know the old saying "I can lose weight but you will always be ugly" usually referring to the persons inner being. Well, there is a solution, in order to make permanent any weight loss, we need to make physical changes to our bodies, that have been built over generations. The use of gastric bands as a method for weight loss has been a significant development in the field of bariatric surgery, providing a minimally invasive option for individuals struggling with severe obesity. Gastric bands, also known as laparoscopic adjustable gastric bands (LAGB), are designed to help patients lose weight by limiting the amount of food they can consume and promoting a feeling of fullness with smaller portions. This surgical intervention has been particularly valuable for those who have not found success with traditional weight loss methods such as diet and exercise.

The history of gastric band surgery is rooted in the broader evolution of bariatric procedures. The concept of restrictive weight loss surgery dates back to the 1970s and 1980s when surgeons began exploring less invasive alternatives to the more complex and permanent gastric bypass procedures. The goal was to develop a method that would be both effective and reversible, allowing patients to manage their weight without the same level of surgical risk or long-term commitment associated with bypass surgeries.

Governments are increasingly turning to gastric bypass surgery to combat obesity due to its effectiveness in preventing long-term health complications. Obesity is linked to numerous chronic conditions, including type 2 diabetes, cardiovascular disease, and certain cancers, which place a significant financial burden on healthcare systems. By addressing obesity surgically, governments aim to reduce the prevalence of these conditions and, consequently, lower healthcare costs over time.

Countries like the United Kingdom and France offer gastric bypass surgery free of charge through their public healthcare systems. In these nations, the surgery is available not only to adults but also to younger individuals struggling with severe obesity, recognising the importance of early intervention. This proactive approach is seen as a viable financial strategy, as preventing obesity-related diseases can significantly reduce long-term healthcare expenditure.

Gastric bypass surgery is intended to prevent several conditions prevalent in older populations. These include type 2 diabetes, which often requires costly long-term treatment and can lead to complications like neuropathy and kidney disease. Cardiovascular diseases, including heart attacks and strokes, are also common among obese individuals and result in substantial medical costs. Additionally, obesity is a major risk factor for osteoarthritis, which can severely impair mobility and quality of life in older adults, further increasing healthcare spending on treatments and surgeries.

Evidence supporting the cost-effectiveness of gastric bypass surgery is robust. A study published in The Lancet found that bariatric surgery, including gastric bypass, significantly reduces the incidence of type 2 diabetes and cardiovascular events. Moreover, a report from the National Health Service (NHS) in the UK highlighted that the upfront costs of gastric bypass surgery are offset within 2-4 years due to reduced expenditure on obesity-related conditions.

By offering gastric bypass surgery, governments aim to address obesity proactively, reducing the long-term burden on healthcare systems and improving the health and quality of life of their populations. This strategy not only addresses immediate health concerns but also ensures sustainable healthcare expenditure in the future.

Adjustable Gastric Band (LAP-BAND)

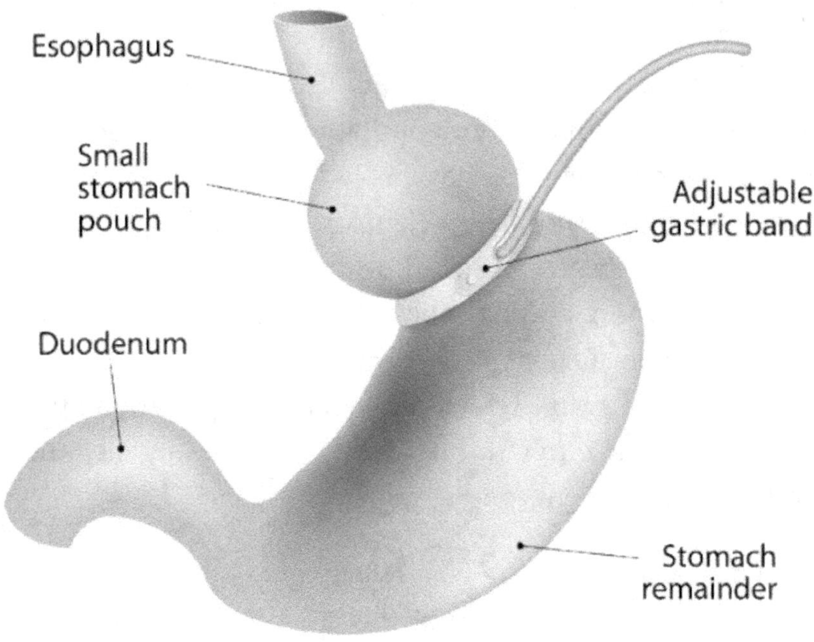

The modern gastric band, as we know it today, was significantly developed by the Swedish company Allergan (formerly Inamed Health), which introduced the LAP-BAND system. This system gained approval from the U.S. Food and Drug Administration (FDA) in 2001, marking a significant milestone in the availability of weight loss surgeries. Another notable product is the REALIZE Band, developed by Ethicon Endo-Surgery, a subsidiary of Johnson & Johnson, which received FDA approval in 2007. These devices consist of a silicone ring that can be adjusted by inflating or deflating a balloon inside the band through a port placed under the skin. This adjustability is a key feature, as it allows for the band to be tightened or loosened based on the patient's progress and needs, thereby controlling the size of the stomach pouch and the rate at which food passes through it.

The surgical procedure to fit a gastric band is typically performed laparoscopically, involving several small incisions in the abdomen. Through these incisions, a camera and surgical instruments are inserted, allowing the surgeon to place the band around the upper part of the stomach and secure it in position. The port, which is used for adjustments, is attached to the abdominal wall and accessed with a needle to add or remove saline from the band's inner balloon.

Surgeons performing gastric band procedures must possess specialised training and certification in bariatric surgery. This training includes comprehensive knowledge of anatomy, specific techniques for placing and adjusting the band, and the management of potential complications. Surgeons typically undergo rigorous training, including residency and fellowship programs in bariatric surgery, and must meet the standards set by professional organisations such as the American Society for Metabolic and Bariatric Surgery (ASMBS) or the British Obesity and Metabolic Surgery Society (BOMSS).

Clinical trials and studies have been instrumental in establishing the efficacy and safety of gastric bands for weight loss. One of the landmark studies in this area was published in the Annals of Surgery in 2003, which followed 500 patients over three years and reported an average excess weight loss of 47%. Another significant study, published in Obesity Surgery in 2004, found that patients experienced significant improvements in obesity-related conditions, such as type 2 diabetes, hypertension, and sleep apnoea, following gastric band surgery.

Despite these promising early results, the use of gastric bands has been subject to ongoing scrutiny and debate. Long-term studies have revealed a more nuanced picture of their efficacy and safety. For instance, a study published in JAMA Surgery in 2011 followed patients for up to 10 years and found that while many achieved substantial weight loss, a significant number experienced complications or required additional surgeries to address issues such as band slippage, erosion, or infection. This highlighted the importance of careful patient selection and long-term follow-up.

Further research, including a systematic review and meta-analysis published in 2014 in Surgery for Obesity and Related Diseases, concluded that gastric bands were effective for weight loss and improvement of comorbid conditions but emphasised the need for careful patient selection and long-term follow-up. This study underscored that the success of the procedure is heavily influenced by the patient's adherence to lifestyle changes and regular medical monitoring.

Statistics on the number of gastric bands fitted in developed nations indicate a fluctuating trend. In the United States, the peak of gastric band surgeries occurred in the mid-2000s, with estimates suggesting that over 35,000 procedures were performed annually during that period. However, the numbers have since declined, partly due to the rise of alternative bariatric procedures like sleeve gastrectomy and gastric bypass, which have shown higher success rates and fewer complications in some studies. In the United Kingdom, the National Health Service (NHS) has provided gastric band surgery as part of its weight management services for eligible patients. Data from the

NHS indicates that several thousand gastric band procedures were performed annually in the early 2010s. However, like in the United States, the popularity of the procedure has waned in favour of other surgical options.

The impact of gastric bands on patients' lives is multifaceted, extending beyond mere weight loss. Numerous anecdotal accounts highlight the transformative effects of the surgery. Celebrities and public figures have occasionally shared their experiences with gastric bands, contributing to public awareness and acceptance of the procedure. For instance, former reality TV star Sharon Osbourne publicly discussed her decision to undergo gastric band surgery in the early 2000s. She attributed her significant weight loss to the procedure and spoke candidly about the challenges and benefits of living with a gastric band.

Similarly, comedian and actress Roseanne Barr underwent gastric band surgery in 1998 and experienced notable weight loss. She has spoken about how the surgery helped her manage her weight more effectively and improve her overall health. These high-profile endorsements have undoubtedly played a role in shaping public perception of gastric bands as a viable weight loss solution.

However, it is important to acknowledge that gastric band surgery is not a one-size-fits-all solution. The variability in patient outcomes underscores the need for thorough preoperative evaluation and patient education. Candidates for gastric band surgery typically undergo a comprehensive assessment to determine their suitability for the procedure. This includes evaluating their medical history, psychological readiness, and commitment to making the necessary lifestyle changes to ensure long-term success.

In addition to the initial surgery, patients require ongoing follow-up care to monitor their progress and make necessary adjustments to the band. Regular consultations with a multidisciplinary team, including surgeons, dietitians, and psychologists, are crucial for addressing any complications and supporting patients in achieving their weight loss goals.

The future of gastric band surgery continues to evolve as new technologies and techniques emerge. Advances in minimally invasive surgery and improved band designs aim to enhance the safety and efficacy of the procedure. Additionally, ongoing research seeks to identify patient characteristics that predict successful outcomes, enabling more personalised and targeted interventions.

While gastric band surgery remains a valuable option for weight loss, it is essential to consider it within the broader context of comprehensive weight management strategies. Combining surgical interventions with behavioural therapy, nutritional counselling, and physical activity is crucial for achieving sustained weight loss and improving overall health outcomes.

The use of gastric bands for weight loss has a rich history marked by innovation, clinical trials, and real-world experiences. Developed as a less invasive alternative to other bariatric procedures, gastric bands have helped many individuals achieve significant weight loss and improve their health. However, the procedure is not without risks, and careful patient selection, thorough preoperative evaluation, and ongoing follow-up care are essential for maximising its benefits.

As medical science continues to advance, the future of gastric band surgery holds promise for further improving outcomes and providing effective weight loss solutions for those in need.

Gastric bypass surgery, also known as Roux-en-Y gastric bypass, and gastric stapling, including procedures like vertical banded gastroplasty, represent significant advancements in the field of bariatric surgery. These procedures are designed to facilitate substantial weight loss in individuals with severe obesity, especially when other weight loss methods have proven ineffective. While both gastric bypass and stapling surgeries aim to reduce food intake and promote weight loss, they employ different techniques and mechanisms to achieve these goals.

Gastric bypass surgery is a complex procedure that involves creating a small pouch at the top of the stomach and then connecting this pouch directly to the small intestine, effectively bypassing a significant portion of the stomach and the first part of the small intestine (duodenum). This results in two primary mechanisms for weight loss: restriction and malabsorption. The restricted stomach pouch limits the amount of food that can be consumed at one time, while the bypassed section of the intestine reduces the number of calories and nutrients absorbed from food.

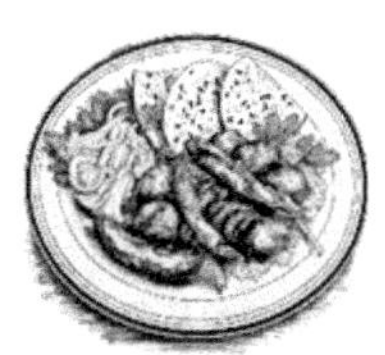

GASTRIC BYPASS

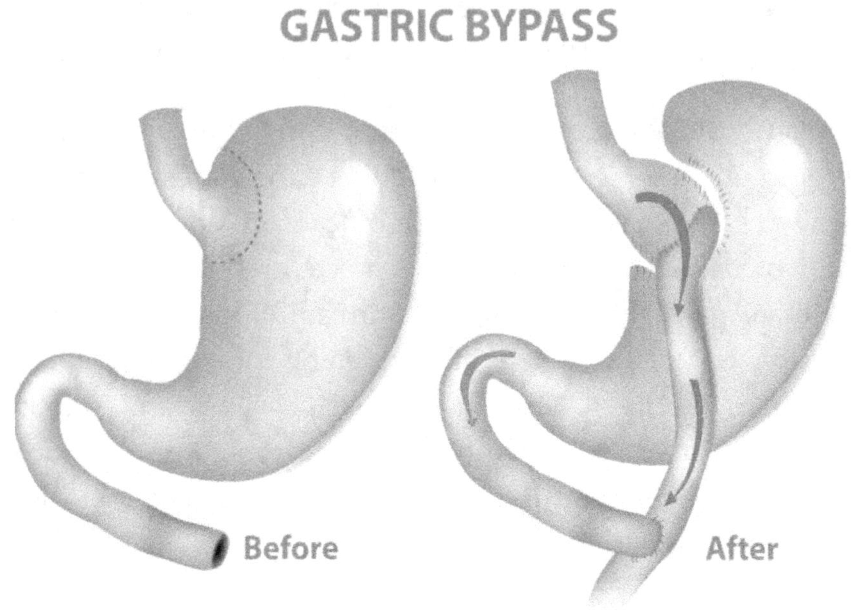

The history of gastric bypass surgery dates back to the 1960s when Dr. Edward Mason, often regarded as the "father of obesity surgery," developed the first gastric bypass procedure. Dr. Mason's pioneering work laid the foundation for modern bariatric surgery and highlighted the potential of surgical interventions in the treatment of obesity. Over the years, the technique has evolved significantly, with improvements in surgical methods and patient care leading to better outcomes and reduced risks.

In contrast to gastric bypass, gastric stapling procedures focus primarily on restricting the size of the stomach without altering the digestive tract's normal flow. Vertical banded gastroplasty (VBG), one of the earliest and most common forms of gastric stapling, involves creating a small stomach pouch using surgical staples and reinforcing it with a band to prevent stretching. This procedure was developed in the 1980s by Dr. Edward Mason and Dr. Chikashi Itoh as an alternative to more invasive bariatric surgeries.

Gastric bypass and stapling surgeries require specialised equipment and training. Surgeons performing these procedures must be skilled in advanced laparoscopic techniques and have a thorough understanding of bariatric principles. They typically undergo extensive training, including general surgery residency and additional fellowship training in bariatric surgery. Professional organisations such as the American Society for Metabolic and Bariatric Surgery (ASMBS) and the British Obesity and Metabolic Surgery Society (BOMSS) provide certification and accreditation for bariatric surgeons, ensuring high standards of care.

Clinical trials and studies have played a crucial role in establishing the efficacy and safety of gastric bypass and stapling surgeries. The landmark Swedish Obese Subjects (SOS) study, initiated in 1987, is one of the most comprehensive and long-term studies examining the effects of bariatric surgery, including gastric bypass. The study followed over 4,000 participants for more than two decades and found that those who underwent bariatric surgery, including gastric bypass, experienced significant and sustained weight loss compared to those who received conventional treatment. Additionally, the study reported improvements in obesity-related conditions such as type 2 diabetes, cardiovascular disease, and mortality rates.

Another significant study, published in the New England Journal of Medicine in 2007, compared the outcomes of gastric bypass surgery with those of non-surgical weight loss methods.

The results showed that gastric bypass patients achieved greater and more sustained weight loss, with an average loss of 31% of their initial body weight after 10 years. Moreover, the surgery led to substantial improvements in quality of life and obesity-related comorbidities.

Gastric bypass surgery has become one of the most commonly performed bariatric procedures worldwide. In the United States, it is estimated that over 200,000 bariatric surgeries are performed annually, with gastric bypass accounting for a significant portion of these procedures. In the United Kingdom, the National Health Service (NHS) has provided gastric bypass surgery as part of its weight management services for eligible patients, with thousands of procedures performed each year.

Celebrities and public figures have often turned to gastric bypass surgery to address their weight issues, bringing public attention to the procedure. One notable example is the American television personality Al Roker, who underwent gastric bypass surgery in 2002. Roker has been open about his weight loss journey, crediting the surgery for helping him lose over 100 pounds and improve his health. His experience has inspired many others to consider surgical options for weight loss.

Similarly, British singer-songwriter and television personality Sharon Osbourne underwent gastric bypass surgery in 1999. Osbourne has spoken candidly about her struggles with weight and how the surgery helped her achieve a healthier lifestyle. Her story, like many others, highlights the potential of gastric bypass surgery to transform lives and improve overall well-being.

Despite the success stories, it is essential to recognise that gastric bypass and stapling surgeries are not without risks and complications. Common complications include nutritional deficiencies, infections, and gastrointestinal issues. Long-term follow-up care is crucial to monitor patients' health and address any complications promptly. Patients must adhere to strict dietary guidelines and take vitamin and mineral supplements to prevent deficiencies.

Gastric bypass and stapling surgeries represent significant advancements in the treatment of obesity, offering hope to individuals struggling with severe weight issues. These procedures, developed and refined over decades, have demonstrated their efficacy in achieving substantial and sustained weight loss, improving quality of life, and reducing obesity-related comorbidities. As medical science continues to advance, these surgeries will likely become even safer and more effective, providing a valuable tool in the fight against obesity.

Finally, the other solution are the recent developments and advances in weight loss drugs; Ozempic, known chemically as semaglutide, has gained considerable attention in recent years for its effectiveness in weight management. Originally developed and marketed by Novo Nordisk, a Danish multinational pharmaceutical company, Ozempic was primarily designed to treat type 2 diabetes. However, its potential as a weight loss drug has since become a significant point of interest within the medical community and beyond.

The development of Ozempic began in the laboratories of Novo Nordisk, where scientists aimed to create a medication to improve glycaemic control in diabetic patients. Semaglutide, the active ingredient in Ozempic, is a glucagon-like peptide-1

(GLP-1) receptor agonist. GLP-1 is a hormone that stimulates insulin secretion in response to meals, thereby lowering blood sugar levels. Semaglutide mimics this hormone, enhancing insulin release while also suppressing glucagon, a hormone that raises blood sugar levels.

The development of semaglutide was a significant scientific breakthrough. Its ability to withstand degradation by enzymes in the digestive system, unlike earlier GLP-1 analogues, meant it could be administered via injection once a week. This marked a notable improvement in patient compliance compared to the daily injections required by other GLP-1 receptor agonists. Ozempic was approved for medical use in the United States by the Food and Drug Administration (FDA) in December 2017 and by the European Medicines Agency (EMA) shortly thereafter. Initially, it was marketed solely as a treatment for type 2 diabetes. However, early clinical observations hinted at an unexpected benefit: significant weight loss among patients.

The potential of Ozempic as a weight loss drug spurred a series of rigorous clinical trials to evaluate its efficacy and safety in non-diabetic individuals with obesity. The STEP (Semaglutide Treatment Effect in People with obesity) programme was a pivotal series of trials that focused on this new application. The STEP 1 trial, a 68-week study involving nearly 2,000 participants, demonstrated remarkable results. Participants receiving 2.4 mg of semaglutide weekly lost an average of 14.9% of their body weight compared to just 2.4% in the placebo group. The STEP 2 trial, involving individuals with type 2 diabetes, also showed significant weight loss, though to a lesser degree than the non-diabetic cohort. These results were replicated in subsequent trials, such as STEP 3 and STEP 4, which further established semaglutide's efficacy in weight management. Notably, the STEP 3 trial, which incorporated intensive behavioural therapy alongside semaglutide, showed even greater weight reduction, underscoring the benefits of a multifaceted approach to weight loss.

In 2021, the FDA approved semaglutide for chronic weight management under the brand name Wegovy. This marked a significant milestone, positioning semaglutide as a dual-purpose drug for both diabetes management and obesity treatment. Since its approval, numerous studies have sought to explore the broader impacts of semaglutide on weight loss and overall health. A comprehensive review published in The Lancet in 2022 synthesised data from several trials, concluding that semaglutide not only promoted weight loss but also improved cardiovascular health markers. This included reductions in waist circumference, blood pressure, and levels of C-reactive protein, an inflammation marker linked to cardiovascular risk.

Moreover, a study in the New England Journal of Medicine in 2021 highlighted semaglutide's potential to improve quality of life. Participants reported better physical functioning, higher energy levels, and greater overall satisfaction with their weight loss journey. Beyond clinical trials, real-world data has also underscored semaglutide's effectiveness. A large-scale observational study involving over 20,000 patients found that those prescribed semaglutide experienced significant weight loss, with many achieving a weight reduction of 10% or more. This study, conducted across multiple countries, provided robust evidence supporting semaglutide's role in weight management outside the controlled environment of clinical trials.

The rising popularity of semaglutide as a weight loss drug has inevitably attracted attention from high-profile individuals and celebrities. Although specific endorsements are often kept under wraps due to privacy and ethical considerations, several anecdotes suggest its widespread use among the elite. One notable example is the rumoured use by various Hollywood celebrities, who have purportedly turned to semaglutide to achieve rapid weight loss for film roles or red-carpet events. While these claims are often speculative, the allure of a scientifically backed, highly effective weight loss solution is undoubtedly appealing in industries where physical appearance can significantly impact career opportunities.

Furthermore, social media influencers have also played a role in popularising semaglutide. Several high-profile fitness and wellness influencers have shared their weight loss journeys on platforms like Instagram and YouTube, crediting semaglutide for their dramatic transformations. These personal testimonials, though anecdotal, have contributed to the drug's growing reputation as a potent weight loss aid.

To understand why semaglutide is effective for weight loss, it is essential to delve into its mechanism of action. Semaglutide's primary function is to mimic the GLP-1 hormone, which has several physiological effects that contribute to weight loss. Firstly, it slows gastric emptying, leading to prolonged satiety after meals. This results in reduced caloric intake as individuals feel full for longer periods. Secondly, semaglutide acts on the brain's appetite centres, reducing hunger and food cravings. This central action is particularly significant as it addresses the neurological aspect of eating behaviour, making it easier for individuals to adhere to a reduced-calorie diet. Lastly, semaglutide promotes insulin secretion in response to elevated blood glucose levels, improving glycaemic control. This dual action of enhancing insulin sensitivity and reducing appetite makes it a valuable tool for both diabetes management and weight loss.

Like any medication, semaglutide is not without its side effects. The most commonly reported adverse effects are gastrointestinal in nature, including nausea, vomiting, and diarrhoea. These symptoms are usually transient and tend to diminish over time as the body adjusts to the medication. More severe, albeit rare, side effects include pancreatitis and gallbladder disease. Consequently, patients with a history of these conditions are generally advised to avoid semaglutide. Thyroid C-cell tumours have been observed in rodent studies, although no conclusive evidence has linked semaglutide to thyroid cancer in humans. Nonetheless, patients with a personal or family history of medullary thyroid carcinoma or Multiple Endocrine Neoplasia syndrome type 2 are contraindicated from using the drug. Due to these potential risks, healthcare providers typically conduct thorough evaluations before prescribing semaglutide, ensuring it is appropriate for the individual's health profile. Additionally, ongoing monitoring is recommended to detect and manage any adverse effects promptly.

The success of semaglutide has sparked interest in the development of next-generation GLP-1 receptor agonists with even greater efficacy and fewer side effects. Novo Nordisk and other pharmaceutical companies are actively exploring new formulations and combinations with other weight loss agents to enhance therapeutic outcomes. One such promising development is the investigation of oral semaglutide formulations, which could offer a more convenient alternative to injections. Early trials have shown encouraging results, suggesting that oral semaglutide may be similarly effective for weight management. Furthermore, research is ongoing to understand the long-term impacts of semaglutide on metabolic health, cardiovascular outcomes, and overall mortality. These studies will provide valuable insights into the broader benefits and potential risks associated with prolonged use.

The growing popularity of semaglutide as a weight loss drug also raises important ethical and societal considerations. The high cost of the medication, particularly in regions without robust healthcare coverage, poses a significant barrier to access for many individuals. This disparity underscores the need for policies that ensure equitable access to effective weight loss treatments. Additionally, the marketing of semaglutide and similar drugs must be handled with care to avoid promoting unrealistic body image standards or fostering a culture of quick-fix solutions to weight management. Public health campaigns should emphasise the importance of a holistic approach to weight loss, incorporating diet, exercise, and behavioural modifications alongside pharmacological interventions.

Ozempic, or semaglutide, represents a significant advancement in the field of weight management, offering a powerful tool for individuals struggling with obesity. Its journey from a diabetes medication to a widely recognised weight loss drug underscores the potential of scientific innovation to address complex health challenges. While the drug's efficacy is well-documented, ongoing research and careful consideration of ethical implications are essential to maximise its benefits and ensure it is accessible to all who may benefit from its use. As we look to the future, the continued evolution of weight loss pharmacotherapy promises to bring new hope to millions, transforming lives and improving health outcomes on a global scale. Through a combination of cutting-edge science, thoughtful regulation, and equitable healthcare policies, the promise of semaglutide can be fully realised, offering a brighter, healthier future for those battling obesity.

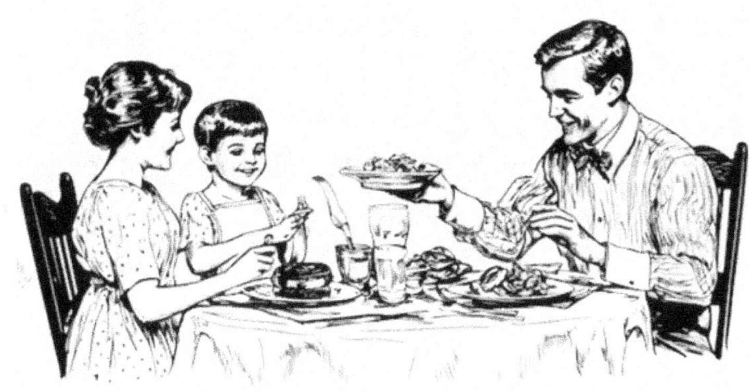

AUTHORS EPILOGUE

As we reach the end of "How Long Does it Take, To Make, A Fat Person?" I hope you have gained valuable insights into the intricate interplay between genetics, history, and environment in shaping human body size and composition. This journey through time and across cultures has shown us that our bodies are a testament to the resilience and adaptability of our species.

Throughout this book, we have explored how centuries of food scarcity in regions like China and Ireland have sculpted genetic predispositions, and how recent changes in food availability have led to rapid increases in obesity rates. These case studies underscore the profound impact that environmental factors have on our bodies, revealing that while individual lifestyle choices are important, they are often overshadowed by our genetic heritage and historical context.

For young readers on the cusp of higher education, I hope this book has provided a deeper appreciation of our species' remarkable adaptability. Understanding the genetic and environmental factors that determine body size and shape can help us move beyond simplistic notions of willpower and discipline. It is crucial to acknowledge that shaming individuals for their body type is not only unjust but also ignores the complex factors at play.

As we look to the future, I propose some solutions for achieving and maintaining a healthy weight within our lifetimes. However, I recognise that this is just the beginning. I hope this book inspires budding young scientists to take this research further, uncovering more secrets of human adaptability and working towards a healthier, more understanding world.

So finally, and to answer my own question, it is my firm belief that it takes 6 generations at least to change a heretical body plan, whether that is going from a famine starved individual to an obese person, and similarly 6 generations from an obese family to a family that all have what is taken today as a healthy weight. However as stated that is not to say that you can make all of the personal sacrifices like attending the gym every day, and living on salads, but it will always be a struggle.

In conclusion, let us embrace our diversity and learn from our past. Our differences are a testament to the strength and resilience of our species. By supporting each other and promoting understanding, we can work towards a future where everyone can achieve their healthiest selves. Thank you for joining me on this enlightening journey through history, genetics, and human resilience.

Bibliography

Encyclopaedia Britannica

How We Got to Now; by Steven Johnson

Our Human Story Paperback –by Louise Humphrey and Chris Stringer

The Dawn of Everything by David Graeber & David Wengrow

The Evolution of Everything by Matt Ridley

The World A Brief Introduction by Richard Haass

Roseboom, T. J., et al. (2001). "Effects of prenatal exposure to the Dutch famine on adult disease in later life: an overview." Molecular and Cellular Endocrinology.

Heijmans, B. T., et al. (2008). "Persistent epigenetic differences associated with prenatal exposure to famine in humans." Proceedings of the National Academy of Sciences.

Lumey, L. H., Stein, A. D., & Susser, E. (2011). "Prenatal famine and adult health." Annual Review of Public Health.

O'Rahilly, S., & Farooqi, I. S. (2008). "Human obesity: a heritable neurobehavioral disorder that is highly sensitive to environmental conditions." Diabetes.

Weaver, I. C., et al. (2004). "Epigenetic programming by maternal behavior." Nature Neuroscience.

Diamond, J. (2001). "Unhealed wounds: Reflections on the Dutch Hunger Winter." Nature.

Lomolino, M. V. (2005). "Body size evolution in insular vertebrates: generality of the island rule." Journal of Biogeography.

Van der Knaap, W. P. (1996). "Palaeoloxodon falconeri: the dwarf elephant of Sicily." Mammal Review.

Hewlett, B. S., & Lamb, M. E. (2005). "Hunter-gatherer childhoods: Evolutionary, developmental, and cultural perspectives." Transaction Publishers.

Thank you for choosing this book

Please consider leaving a review on Amazon:

Please share this QR code with a friend or family.

Statistically only one in every two hundred readers take the time to write a review, so if you enjoyed this offering, please consider writing one it really helps the author.

https://www.amazon.com/dp/B0DBNXDDBP